Cut Down

Cut Down to Size covers everything you need to know about bariatric surgery, from referral through to the challenges you may face after surgery. Most people who seek weight loss surgery have struggled for many years to control their eating, and have experienced increasing ill health, self-consciousness and discrimination. People see weight loss surgery as their last chance for a better, more normal, life. While hopeful fantasies about an alternative future make it hard to contemplate the risk of failure, some patients experience considerable emotional or physical problems.

This book offers insight into the realities of living with weight loss surgery, and practical exercises help you think through your emotional readiness, social circumstances and eating habits that could determine the success of surgery. Active preparation for surgery by making psychological and lifestyle changes puts you in the best position to achieve better health and emotional well-being.

Cut Down to Size is the first book to focus on the psychological and social aspects of weight loss surgery and will be of interest to health professionals as well as anyone contemplating weight loss surgery. By sharing the experiences of other bariatric patients, the reader can appreciate the nature of life after surgery and make a judgement about their capacity to cope with these demands.

Jenny Radcliffe is a Consultant Clinical Health Psychologist. Since completing her training at University College London she has specialised in working with people with physical health problems. For the past eight years her primary interest has been in the psychological impact of obesity and weight loss surgery.

Cut Down to Size
Achieving success with weight loss surgery

Jenny Radcliffe

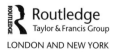

Routledge
Taylor & Francis Group

LONDON AND NEW YORK

First published 2013
by Routledge
2 Park Square, Milton Park, Abingdon, Oxon OX14 4RN

Simultaneously published in the USA and Canada
by Routledge
711 Third Avenue, New York, NY 10017

Routledge is an imprint of the Taylor & Francis Group, an informa business

British Library Cataloguing in Publication Data
A catalogue record for this book is available from the British Library

Library of Congress Cataloging in Publication Data
A catalog record for this book has been requested

ISBN: 978-0-415-68376-0 (hbk)
ISBN: 978-0-415-68377-7 (pbk)
ISBN: 978-0-203-07469-5 (ebk)

Typeset in New Century Schoolbook
by RefineCatch Limited, Bungay, Suffolk

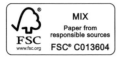

Printed and bound by CPI Group (UK) Ltd, Croydon, CR0 4YY

This book is dedicated to my wonderful daughters Niamh and Molly.

Contents

Illustrations

Preface

When I first started working with bariatric patients in 2003, I was struck by the complexity of the decision they faced; whether to undergo potentially life-threatening surgery for the elusive promise of a happier life. In my previous work, patients suffering from chronic back pain, cancer and heart disease had also faced immense social and emotional challenges as the result of ill-health and disability, their family and work lives often devastated by their health problems. But somehow the patients I was now seeing, referred by surgeons to determine whether they were 'psychologically suitable' for weight loss surgery, seemed to confront a quite different trial, raising issues of personal control and responsibility, the power of medicine and the nature of our relationship with food as a source of pleasure and comfort.

Media representations of obesity and weight loss surgery present a mix of joy and horror. A celebrity's shrinking form documented by the weekly magazines; a woman who sells her house to pay for surgery to remove excess skin; a man finding love after losing half his body weight; a woman charging men to watch her eat online so she can raise the money for bariatric surgery; whether portrayed as a magical cure or medically endorsed mutilation designed to force people into a socially acceptable norm, weight loss surgery is rarely viewed objectively. For many patients surgery is seen as offering hope of escape from a life defined by their weight. It is seen as something that can be attained only if you can prove yourself worthy; so patients make supplication to those who hold the key – the primary care trust (PCT) fund-holders and surgeons who decide who will, and who will not, be granted this new beginning. With the promise of a magical cure, patients often close their eyes to the reality of living with weight loss surgery; what it can offer, what it can't and what they must do to achieve success.

After seeing someone for assessment I would often feel they simply didn't know enough about the pros and cons to make a reasoned decision. As driven as they were to change their lives, patients put little thought into what this would involve or how they might feel as they see themselves shrinking in size. They would often talk about avoiding any 'negative' information – the risks and complications that might cause them to reconsider their decision – and rarely reflected on any emotional downside. I would find myself at the end of the meeting encouraging my client to go away, do more research and think hard about the commitment they were making – that they would never again be able to rely on food for commiseration or celebration in a way they took for granted. Understandably my clients asked me where they should look for this information and that's where I got stuck. There didn't seem to be a straightforward comprehensive guide that could lead them through this process. Many of the books already available were from the USA and had a strong state-side slant, including lots of information about how to persuade your health insurer to pay. While some of these books covered the procedures and the medical risks well, they paid little attention to the psychological side of weight loss surgery. Many of the books were little more than cookery books and offered no advice to those patients who continued to struggle to control their eating. None seemed to mention the possibility of failure. The internet wasn't much better; hundreds of websites offered information about surgery of variable quality and often with a strong positive bias (particularly in those selling weight loss surgery services). On the other hand, there were chat rooms with accounts of people's individual experiences but these were polarised, often either very positive or very negative. I'm very much in favour of would-be patients hearing about the lives of people who have had surgery and always encourage them to attend a support group before they make a final decision, but these personal stories needed to be balanced against a robust understanding of the facts of surgery – the knowledge that has been amassed from hundreds of scientific studies.

So I decided to write this book to fill the gap for a guide to the physical and emotional impact of bariatric surgery. Knowing what life will be like after weight loss surgery is rather like knowing what life will be like after you have a child. You've heard the warnings of sleepless nights and restrictions on your freedom, but you focus on the upsides – of which there are many – hoping the rest will work itself out. This book is like a book about parenthood; it will not enable you to avoid all challenges, but at least you'll be better at recognising them when they come along and may have some strategies in hand for coping with them. I hope this book will be a helpful guide as you take your weight loss surgery, enabling you to bypass some of the stumbling blocks and navigate those that you can't dodge. I wish you well in your journey and hope you arrive where you want to be.

Acknowledgements

I would like to offer my heartfelt gratitude to my colleagues in the bariatric services at St George's Healthcare NHS Trust, Ashford and St Peters Hospitals NHS Foundation Trust with particular thanks to Mr Marcus Reddy and Mr Samer Humadi, Dr Tom Stevens and Scott Lonnee. Also to Adrian Weston for his generously offered professional advice; Gary Rimmer for his robust feedback and tenacious encouragement; Leo Estall and Sophie Doswell for their time, thoughts and encouragement; Guy Brown for his guidance and being a lovely brother-in-law; Carol Bowen Ball for putting me in touch with the weight loss surgery patients who shared their experiences with me so generously; Imperial College Healthcare NHS Trust for kindly giving permission to use their illustrations; Joanne Forshaw at Routledge for offering me this opportunity; Versha Talati for tolerating my occasional distractedness; Richard Stantiford for his input on the role of exercise; Ernie Govier for his faith, support and encouragement over many years; Donald and my daughters for their endless patience; and finally to the bariatric patients who I have worked with over the years – I wish you all well.

Abbreviations

BMI	body mass index
BPD/DS	biliopancreatic diversion/duodenal switch
CBT	cognitive-behavioural therapy
CPAP	continuous positive airway pressure
DVT	deep-vein thrombosis
EWL	excess weight loss
GORD	gastro-oesophageal reflux disease
LAGB	laparoscopic adjustable gastric band
NAFLD	non-alcoholic fatty liver disease
NES	night eating syndrome
NICE	National Institute for Health and Clinical Excellence
NPY	neuropeptide Y
NSAIDs	non-steroidal anti-inflammatory drugs
OSA	obstructive sleep apnoea
PCOS	polycystic ovary syndrome
PCT	primary care trust
PE	pulmonary emboli
RMR	resting metabolic rate
RYGB	Roux-en-Y gastric bypass
TIA	transient ischaemic attack
VPAP	variable positive airway pressure

The obesity epidemic and weight loss surgery

People seeking weight loss surgery are at the end of the line. They have tried all the conventional means of losing weight; they have attended Weight Watchers, Slimming World, Rosemary Conley; they have eaten cabbage, eggs and grapefruits, high protein, low fat, low carbs, no carbs; they have bought CDs from Paul McKenna, milkshakes from LighterLife and tablets over the internet. Many have spent thousands of pounds on their attempts to lose weight but remain obese. They might have lost a substantial amount of weight before it creeps back on and the cycle of hope and despair continues. At some point, when they cannot face another diet failure, they ask their GP to be referred for weight loss surgery, seeing it as a foolproof means of controlling the uncontrollable. Once they have funding and are sitting in front of the surgeon, they face an avalanche of medical information. Heightened anxiety, poor understanding, denial of risks and hopeful fantasies about their alternative future all contribute to people's difficulty in making a thoughtful decision.

Do you recognise yourself or a loved one in the description above? Have you been referred or are you thinking about weight loss surgery as an option? This book is written to help you make the best decision you can. It will provide you with detailed information about the process from referral to post-surgery lifestyle changes. Over the course of this book you will be able to build up a clear picture of the challenges of weight loss surgery, embracing practical information about the different procedures, their risks and difficulties and the real experiences of weight loss surgery patients, both successful and unsuccessful. Practical exercises assess your suitability for surgery, help you reflect on your social and emotional resources and prepare you for the changes you will face. By working through this book, hearing about the lessons learnt by others and considering your own situation, you will be in the best position to make an informed decision.

Obesity is not an individual problem, it is a global problem. Worldwide more than *one and a half billion* people[1] are overweight or obese. However much you feel yourself alone with your problem, surrounded by slim people who have no difficulty managing what they eat or controlling their weight, the reality is that obesity is an issue facing increasing numbers of people.

When did the obesity epidemic begin? Scientists differ in their views on this.[2] Was it with the onset of the motor car, TVs and the new supermarkets in the 1940s; the rise of fast food restaurants in the 1970s; or the advent of daytime TV and cheap processed food in the 1980s? Whatever the answer, we are now faced with a problem of obesity at a level never seen before and as you're reading this book, I assume that you or a loved one, or perhaps a client, are part of this epidemic and are wondering whether weight loss surgery is the answer. This book will not only provide you with all the information you need to make an informed decision about weight loss surgery, but will also prepare you for the pitfalls and problems you could encounter after surgery.

The numbers of obese people rose spectacularly between 2000 and 2005. Over this time, in the USA, there was an overall increase in obesity of almost 25 per cent, but a 75 per cent increase in people who are super-morbidly obese. In 2011 the Health and Social Care Information Centre[3] published a report stating that almost a quarter of adults in England are obese (that is, they have a body mass index (BMI) of 30 or more) and another 44 per cent of men and 33 per cent of women are overweight (having a BMI of 25–29). Over a third of the adult population have a raised waist size; when a lot of your weight is carried around your middle it is called *central obesity* and is associated with an increased risk of developing heart problems, metabolic syndrome and diabetes (you can read more about these health problems in Chapter 3). The problem is not restricted to adults; approximately 15 per cent of children between the ages of 2 and 15 are now obese. A government commissioned report by Foresight in 2007[4] predicted that, if no effective action is taken to deal with overweight and obesity, 60 per cent of men, 50 per cent of women and 25 per cent of children would be obese by 2050.

Up to 15 per cent of the population are thought to be at greatly increased risk of health problems, such as diabetes and coronary heart disease, due to their BMI and raised waist measurement[3] and this is why severe overweight is termed morbid obesity. *Morbidity* means health problem so when doctors talk about *morbid obesity* they are not making a judgement about your weight, they are saying that your weight is such that it's likely to affect your health.

The increasing weight of the population, or rather the health problems associated with it, is placing ever greater demands on the health service and the wider economy. It has been estimated that obesity and its health consequences cost the NHS £4.2 billion a year and the economy up to £15 billion in lost productivity.[5] The number of admissions to NHS hospitals of patients with a *primary diagnosis* of obesity (in other words where the doctor felt weight was the main problem) increased over 800 per cent between 1998 and 2009 and almost one and a half million prescriptions for obesity medication were dispensed in 2009, more than 11 times the number of prescriptions in 1999.[3]

Despite growing numbers, severely overweight people are increasingly stigmatised and denigrated. People who are very overweight are seen as deviating from social *rules* about being able to control urges.[6] They have become *the other*, the people it's okay to shout at in the street; seen as weak, even morally deficient, if they just tried harder they could be *thinner, better people*. Obese people are discriminated against socially, educationally and in the workplace[7] and anti-fat attitudes are pervasive across western society. As the average slim person is able lose a kilo or two without too much difficulty, it is assumed that severely overweight people should be able to do the same. Of course losing and maintaining a loss of 10kg is very different from losing 1kg; everyone can hold their breath for one minute, but who can hold it for ten?[8]

Sadly, many obese people internalise these negative attitudes and experience intense distress about their weight and appearance. You may have started to believe these things about yourself – to feel you are weak and out of control and shameful. You may receive little compassion from others and have little sympathy for yourself, making you vulnerable to destructive cycles of over-controlled and uncontrolled eating. The good news is a recent poll in the USA suggested that most people think there should be laws to prevent discrimination on the grounds of weight.[9]

The more a disease is seen as being under the person's control the more social rejection people face.[10] Obesity is viewed by the public as being highly under personal control, and this affects the public view of weight loss surgery. As the disease of obesity is stigmatised, the public do not necessarily want to support and fund medical or surgical treatment for people who are obese.[11] In the context of fat as a *moral failure*, a sign of weak will, people demand that treatments for obesity are harsh and punishing – boot camps and starvation diets. In comparison, weight loss surgery is seen as a *cheat* – an easy way out – and too expensive to be deserved by this devalued group.

The provision of weight loss surgery, both within the NHS and through private health services, has risen dramatically in recent years in response to increasing numbers of people suffering severe weight problems and the failure of current behavioural and dietetic approaches to offer significant and sustained weight loss. As a result of technological advances in surgery, such as keyhole surgery, and improved opportunities for training of surgeons, the balance between the risks of weight loss surgery and the potential benefits has altered dramatically in past decades. As people watch the apparently miraculous changes in the appearance of celebrities who have had weight loss surgery, it's easy to get the impression that the surgeon's knife is a pain-free route to a new life. The reality is that weight loss surgery is not risk free as it can carry considerable physical and psychological challenges, but for some people it can be life changing.

Bariatric surgery

In the 1950s surgeons at the University of Minnesota in the USA, faced with rising numbers of severely overweight patients, wondered whether the weight loss shown after bowel resection could be harnessed as a direct treatment for obesity. The first attempts with intestinal bypass were highly risky, but over the years safe and effective procedures have been developed. Bariatric surgery, from the Greek word *baros* meaning weight, was established. By the 1980s it had become clear that rather than simply producing weight loss, these surgeries also had great benefit for the management of diseases such as type 2 diabetes, high blood pressure and sleep apnoea and, in the USA, the procedures became known as *metabolic and bariatric surgery* to reflect these outcomes.[8]

Bariatrics is the branch of medicine that deals with the causes and treatment of obesity and includes diet, exercise and psychological therapy, as well as medication and surgery. You will hear weight loss surgery called bariatric surgery and the two terms are used interchangeably through this book. Somewhere in the region of 7,000 people had weight loss surgery in the UK in 2009 and 2010,[8] just under 70 per cent through the NHS, 30 per cent privately self-funded and a small proportion paid for through private health insurance. The National Institute for Health and Clinical Excellence (NICE)[12] plan for future services based on the assumption that over a million people have a BMI of over 40 or over 30 with comorbidities, that 60 per cent of these would be considered eligible, and that 40 per cent of these would take up surgery if offered. Within this group it is suggested that around 4,800 could be provided surgery each year, a three-fold increase compared with pre-2007 NHS figures. The same report acknowledged that in 2007 there were almost 50,000 people in England who had a BMI of over 50 and who were, therefore, potentially eligible for weight loss surgery as a *first-line treatment* and that there would be an annual growth in rates of severe obesity of 5 per cent.

The registry of UK bariatric surgery found that a quarter of all bariatric surgery patients had a high level of comorbid disease, including type 2 diabetes and sleep apnoea, and three-quarters had impairment in their day-to-day activities prior to surgery[8] and that these were resolved for around half of all patients one year post-surgery. There is increasing recognition that weight loss surgery can offer savings for the health service. One Canadian study showed that health care costs (including the cost of surgery) were 25 per cent lower in weight loss surgery patients compared with obese people who had not had surgery.[13] It also showed that sick leave and retirement on health grounds decreased five years after surgery.[14]

Given the physical, emotional and social impact of severe overweight, it's understandable that people are increasingly looking to weight loss surgery. With celebrity magazines showing the yo-yoing weight of the rich and famous and revelations that for some the weight was lost through a gastric band or bypass, bariatric surgery has become mainstream. While diets continue to come and go – Dukan, acai berry diet, detox diet, zone diet – people are more aware of the dangers and pitfalls of dieting, with its inbuilt vulnerability to weight cycling and binge eating. Even specialist weight treatments struggle to show good results in the long term. With a conventional weight management programme, 90–95 per cent of participants will have regained all the weight lost within five years.[15] In one study comparing a group of weight loss surgery patients with patients who had been through a weight management programme, the conventional diet and exercise group had an average *gain* of 0.5kg, while the surgery group showed an average 28kg loss over two years[16] together with better outcomes in social and psychological functioning.[17]

Measuring overweight and obesity

The first criterion for weight loss surgery is your weight. When most doctors and scientists talk about weight and obesity they talk about a person's *body mass index* and you will see this referred to throughout the book. The BMI is felt to be the best way to define overweight and obesity, as it is simple to measure and is a reliable way of judging how much body fat people are carrying. Though it has limitations, such as overestimating body fat in people who are very muscular or underestimating body fat in elderly people, it is the most commonly used measure.

Your BMI is a measure of your weight and your height. It can be calculated as weight in kilograms divided by the square of height in metres (kg/m^2). For those of us not numerically gifted, it is easy to find online calculators that will give you your BMI. Doctors may also look at your waist measurement; waist measurement, or the ratio of your waist to your hip (WHR), is sometimes used in combination with BMI as it is a good indicator of elevated health risk.

Table 1.1 Classification of weight by body mass index for adults

BMI score	Classification	Risk of health problems
Less than 18	Underweight	Low
18–24	Healthy weight	Average
25–29	Overweight	Increased
30–34	Obese I	Moderate
35–39	Obese II	Severe
Over 40	Obese III	Very severe

You can see from this chart that people are considered overweight if their BMI is between 25 and 29 and obese if it is over 30. Health risks due to weight increase significantly with a BMI over 35 though even being somewhat overweight is associated with reduced life expectancy.[18]

When it comes to talking about weight a number of different terms are used. People tend to prefer terms such as 'excess weight' and 'weight problem' over excess fat or obesity.[19] *Overweight* and *obese* are *technical* terms based on your BMI; although people sometimes find the word *obese* insulting or upsetting (at times mishearing it as their doctor describing them as 'a beast'), it is a medical term meaning that your weight is such that it carries health risks and is the description most commonly used in medical settings. Other people favour *fat* as it feels more honest or straightforward, but it is not used in this book, except in direct quotes from patients or when talking about fat tissue in the body, as it is often employed in a denigrating or insulting way. The terms very overweight, obese, severe overweight and excessive weight are used largely interchangeably through this book.

Metabolism, eating behaviour and the brain

In the next chapter we will consider some of the factors associated with weight gain in modern day life and you will be able to reflect on your own weight journey, but before you can think about *why* people gain weight, you need to consider *how* people gain weight. You need to know a little about how energy is used by the body and how our brain controls how much you eat.

We all get our energy from food and the energy content in food is measured in terms of *food calories* (kcal). Technically one calorie is the amount of energy required to raise the temperature of one kilogram of water by one degree Celsius. Food – fats, proteins, and carbohydrates and fibre – all release energy during *respiration*, the process by which nutrients are converted into useable energy in the body. Fats and alcohol generate the greatest amount of food energy, followed by proteins and most carbohydrates. Carbohydrates high in fibre are not so easily absorbed and contribute less food energy. The calorie count written on food packaging is calculated by estimating the constituent parts making up the product (protein, carbohydrate, fat and so on) and then converting this to an energy value using standardised tables.

Your resting metabolic rate (RMR) is the amount of energy used for the functioning of vital organs, such as the heart, lungs, kidneys, nervous system, digestive system and so on, while you are at rest. About 70 per cent of calories used each day provide energy for the basic functions of the body. Illness, environmental temperature, exercise and stress levels can affect your RMR. Despite popular belief, people who are overweight do not generally have a slower metabolism than normal weight individuals.

How the brain controls eating[20]

In order to function and stay healthy the body needs to maintain equilibrium between appetite, food intake, energy storage and energy employment. Eating behaviour and energy balance are controlled by a part of the brain called the hypothalamus. Complex interacting signals from the body converge in the hypothalamus, which acts to maintain a state of balance and sustain basic bodily functions.

Although theoretically you can survive for many days or even weeks without food, the reality is that most people tend to think about eating after a few hours without food, and once you've eaten you generally forget about food for a while. Your experience of feeling hungry and feeling full (*satiety*) is the conscious aspect of a series of processes occurring in the body and leading your eating behaviour.

At its most simple, you want to eat when you feel hungry (or possibly before if tempted by the sight or smell of food). Why do you feel hungry? You feel hungry when your stomach and upper intestine are empty; the stomach releases a hormone called *ghrelin* a *hunger hormone* that makes you want to eat. The hypothalamus also detects a fall in insulin levels; decreasing insulin levels are another signal for a need for food. In response to these signals the hypothalamus produces hormones that stimulate hunger and reduce metabolic rate to preserve energy.

Once you've started eating, why do you stop? Again it may seem obvious, but generally you stop eating when you feel full. However the way you feel full is pretty complicated. You get feedback about the nutritional value of food from the mouth and nose as you take in sensory information from tasting and smelling the food. Hormones are released that are sensitive to the nutritional and calorie content of the meal. As you eat your stomach starts to feel distended and the liver sends messages to your brain to say that it is receiving nutrients. Insulin levels rise and ghrelin levels fall, which in turn suppress the production of neurohormones such as *neuropeptide Y* (NPY). Other neurohormones, including peptide YY (PYY), glucose-like peptide-1 (GLP-1) and cholecystokinin (CCK) are released which promote a feeling of fullness and inhibit eating.[21] The chemical messages to keep eating start to be outnumbered by messages to stop eating and you feel full.

Control mechanisms also work to maintain a stable weight over time. When you are well fed, fat cells in the body produce a hormone called *leptin*, which acts on the hypothalamus to suppress the release of hunger hormones. It's the opposite of ghrelin; it acts to inhibit eating and also helps the body use energy to stay warm. When leptin was first discovered, in the 1990s, it was hoped that it could be developed into a medicine to help people lose weight, but most obese people already have high levels of leptin in their system. Instead of having inadequate amounts of leptin it seems that they are *leptin resistant*, the brain is not registering the signal loudly enough. It may be that evolutionary pressure has ensured that rising leptin production in response to increasing fat reserves has only a limited effect on food intake so that people don't restrict their eating to the point of starvation.

So why are so many people becoming overweight? What's happening with these complex mechanisms that should be maintaining a balance between food intake and energy need and keeping our body weight stable? Unfortunately the brain evolved to have a strong mechanism to encourage eating and a disappointingly weak mechanism to inhibit eating. As our ancestors experienced periods of famine, there was always uncertainty about where the next meal would come from, so it made sense that the control mechanisms encouraged people to eat a lot when food was available. Nowadays, when high calorie food is accessible 24/7, many people struggle to control their eating. In the face of high calorie, high reward food the central regulation of energy homeostasis (where energy intake is matched to energy expenditure over time to ensure stability of body fuel) is disrupted. While eating behaviour remains primarily cued by the experience of hunger, there exists on top of this a 'complex network of memories related to eating' (Schweitzer *et al.* 2007: 534)[22] which can compromise the goal of eating to replenish our energy stores (eating to live) and create an urge to eat for pleasure (live to eat).

Tipping the scales

In the real world, away from the laboratory, it is difficult to study the relationship between food intake and energy expenditure in an individual; the number of calories you burn depends on your age, sex, metabolism and activity levels. The recommended daily energy intake values are 2,500 kcal for men and 2,000 kcal for women. Children, older people and people who live sedentary lives need fewer calories and physically active people more. If you eat more calories than you need on a regular basis, you gain weight. Each pound of body fat is made up of around 3,500 calories; if you eat 3,500 calories more than you can use, you'll gain one pound. If you want to lose a pound over one week you need to consume 3,500 calories (about 500 calories a day) less than you need.[23] You don't need to overeat a great deal to be at risk of gaining weight; if you eat just 100 extra calories a day (that is 100 calories that your body doesn't need), the equivalent of a slice of bread or two Jaffa cakes, it adds up to a gain of 4kg in one year.[24]

Fortunately, we are beginning to understand more about the science of obesity. Rather than seeing weight gain as caused simply by uncontrolled greed, there is recognition of the role that modern life and genetics play in the escalating weight of the population. In the next chapter the factors that impact on our ability, or otherwise, to maintain our calorie intake at the correct level will be discussed. These factors, whether environmental, social, psychological or biological invariably affect an aspect of the balance of energy consumed vs. energy expended. You will see how relatively minor alterations in this equilibrium – for example, a satiety signal turned down too low, a genetic tendency to snack, a desire to escape painful feelings, the decision to give up smoking, the start of a new relationship or one more failed diet – can lead to a disruption to the system and the relentless accumulation of additional pounds. By understanding the factors that have contributed to your weight problem you are in the best position to make decisions about how to manage your weight in the future.

As you read this book I hope you will feel more able to understand your personal struggle with weight and the effect on your health and well-being. Chapter 3 outlines the physical and emotional health impact of obesity. Chapter 4 covers the practical aspects of accessing weight loss surgery, as well as helping you think about your personal readiness to make the changes required for successful weight loss. Chapter 5 covers the assessment for surgery; the surgical, dietetic, medical and psychological issues that will be considered by the bariatric team; your expectations of surgery; and the dietary and lifestyle changes you can make to prepare for surgery. Chapter 6 focuses on emotional and practical skills to cope with the demands of surgery, while Chapter 7 provides detailed information about the different surgical procedures including expected weight loss and their risks and benefits. In Chapter 8 the dietary and lifestyle changes you will need to make after surgery are discussed and Chapters 9 and 10 look at people's positive and less happy experiences of surgery respectively. Chapter 11 covers frequently asked questions about weight loss surgery and lists the organisations and websites where you can access support, resources and information. The Further Reading section provides additional information for those of you who wish to follow up any of the studies referred to.

Throughout the book there are practical exercises designed to help you consider your personal suitability for surgery and to support you in developing skills in stress management, self-monitoring, increasing physical activity, assertiveness and problem solving that will help you cope with the demands of surgery and increase the likelihood of a positive outcome. I would encourage you to spend some time on these exercises as you go through the book; they are intended to help you work through the issues of informed consent and access to social and personal resources that are known to play a central role in the success or otherwise of surgery. Remember the decision to proceed with weight loss surgery is only a valid decision if it is likely to lead to a positive outcome for you, that is, the weight loss and improvements in health and emotional well-being need to balance positively against the potential surgical and psychological risks. I hope that, having read this book, you will feel in a better position to be able to judge that balance thoughtfully and realistically.

2

Obesity: a normal response to an abnormal situation?

In Chapter 1 we discussed the complex mechanisms by which the body controls and regulates the balance of energy in (food) and energy out. For thousands of years this delicate system of checks and balances worked pretty well; the majority of the population stayed within healthy weight boundaries. However, in the past 20 years this hard-wired system appears to have stopped functioning effectively. It no longer prevents many of us from regularly consuming too many calories, so more people are becoming overweight or obese and the incidence of weight-related health problems has spiralled upwards. So what's gone wrong?

There are many factors that can affect the balance between energy consumed in calories and energy expended in activity. The factors that influence your vulnerability to becoming overweight (Figure 2.1) work at different levels – environmental, social, psychological and biological – and all these levels can affect each other. For example, hormones released during stress can cause you to gain weight – the psychological level affecting the biological level. If you are depressed you are less likely to motivate yourself to exercise regularly – the psychological level affecting the social level. Or if you have a certain genetic make-up you may have difficulty resisting high calorie foods – the biological level affecting your behaviour.

The following factors can influence your vulnerability to becoming overweight:

- The *obesogenic* (literally obesity-creating) environment we live in today makes you vulnerable to becoming obese because it supplies easily available, cheap and plentiful calories. The environment has also changed in terms of how much physical work you are required to do.

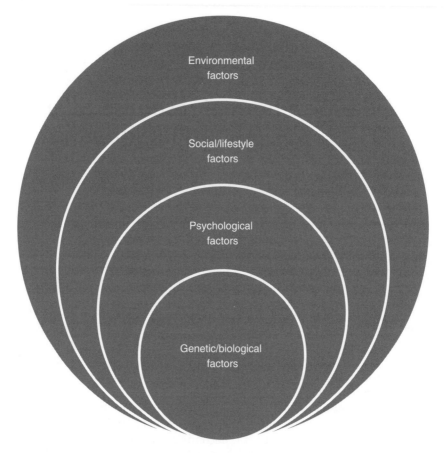

Figure 2.1 Factors that influence your vulnerability to becoming overweight

- Social factors that can impact on weight include changes in lifestyle, life events, the impact of family and relationships, holidays, giving up smoking and opportunity for exercise.
- Psychological factors such as stress, emotional eating, early childhood experiences, eating habits and the impact of failed diet attempts.
- Biological factors, including genetic influences in obesity, the impact of medication, ill health and life stage, are now known to have a major role in weight gain.

This is called a *biopsychosocial* model and it can be used to understand how many different factors act together to alter eating behaviour and vulnerability to obesity. In this chapter you will learn about some of these factors and the ways they have contributed to the increasing weight of the population. You may some recognise some of these from your own life.

Environmental factors: the calorie bonanza

Humans are by nature predisposed to put on weight in response to high availability of energy dense foods and an environment that promotes minimal physical activity. Getting fat has been described as 'a result of a normal response, by normal people, to an abnormal situation' (Swinburn *et al.* 2011).[1]

The most obvious change in the environment over the past 20 years or so is the availability of energy dense (that is, high calorie) and processed foods. In the western world it has never been easier or cheaper to buy calories. You can walk into any supermarket, corner shop or fast food restaurant and buy huge amounts of discounted food. You get to *super-size*, *bogof* and it's all *rolled back*. Supermarkets are so confident in their ability to tempt you to buy more than you need they'll advertise food and drink at a loss just to get you through the door.

As portion sizes have become steadily larger we have become more dependent on external cues when deciding how much to eat. In one great study[2] a *bottomless soup bowl* was designed to refill itself without participants being aware, to show how people use external cues to tell them when to stop eating (*My bowl is empty*) rather than internal cues (*I feel full*). People with the bottomless soup bowl ate more than twice as much as the people eating from normal bowls, but despite this both groups estimated that they had eaten the same number of calories and the bottomless bowl group did not rate themselves as any fuller.

It's not just the cost or availability of food that has changed over the years. There has also been a dramatic change in the *type* of food you can access and the way you eat. We are now able to purchase food 24 hours a day in a variety unknown to previous generations. We lead busy lives with conflicting demands and it's easy to get into the habit of eating on the run or relying on processed, pre-prepared foods. People eat less fresh fruit and vegetables than in their parents' generation and few have the recommended 'five a day'.

If you're anything like the majority of people, you eat on the go and have more snacks. You struggle to keep track of the amount you're eating and may underestimate the calories in the food you eat. Try standing in the queue at the supermarket and picking up some of the snacks on display to check out their calorie count. Some of these small snacks can contain over 500 calories, a quarter of the daily energy need of an adult woman.

Processed foods are often high in fat or sugar (or both) and food manufacturers are well aware of what makes food palatable. Eating foods high in fat, sugar and salt is highly rewarding and the biological goal to replenish energy stores is overridden by a desire to eat for its hedonic (pleasure) value. The stronger the memory of the pleasure value of the food, the stronger the demand for it and the more we want it, the more we'll overeat. Driven by the bombardment of food cues in the environment, these super-delicious foods override the message telling you that you're full and create food cravings[3] so you carry on eating. Your satiety mechanisms are simply not powerful enough to prevent you from overeating in response to such a rewarding experience. It's estimated that calorie consumption has increased by 7 per cent in men and 20 per cent in women since the 1970s.[4]

Opting for diet foods is not the answer. Artificial sweeteners (often found in 'diet', 'lite' and 'low fat' foods and drinks) may also play a role in weight gain. Low-fat labels have been shown to result in people eating around 20 per cent *more* in total calories.[5] Experiments have shown that rats fed yogurt sweetened with a zero-calorie sweetener ate more calories, gained more weight and had higher blood sugar levels than rats fed on sugar-sweetened yogurt.[6] When it comes to humans, one research project studying changes in people's waist

---

Food in the life of a labourer in the eighteenth century

If you were a labourer in the eighteenth century you'd be in good company – they comprised three-quarters of the population. You live in a small rented cottage; your wife and children walk to the communal pump to get water for the family each morning. You leave for work before the sun rises to start your working day, 12 hours hard physical labour, ploughing, sowing, harvesting. You are employed on a daily basis, earning a shilling to support you and your family. Fortunately for you the government set a minimum wage for labourers in 1795, based on the amount of bread your salary could buy. The *Speenhamland allowance* stated that a labourer must be paid the equivalent of 3.72lb of bread a day. You eat only very simple meals; as well as bread, you supplement your diet with potatoes and cabbages you grow in your garden, maybe eggs from your chickens and occasionally meat from the pig you keep on common land.

Food in the eighteenth century was very expensive relative to today. The Speenhamland allowance would be the equivalent of paying around £17.50 for a loaf of bread today. The calorie equivalent of the labourer's wage was around 4,100 calories a day (and that's for the whole family). Nowadays, if you are earning the minimum salary for a nine-hour day you would receive £51.57. Putting aside for a moment the need to budget for housing, clothes, etc. this money could buy you over 15,000 calories, and the variety and deliciousness of the food options available to you now would be unimaginable to the poor eighteenth-century labourer.

measurement over many years, found that people who drank diet fizzy drinks had a 70 per cent greater increase in waist size compared to non-fizzy drink users, even when taking into account physical activity, age, health and so on. People who drank two or more diet fizzy drinks a day showed 500 per cent more increase in waist circumference than non-fizzy drink consumers.[7] One theory is that the mind gets confused when the sweetness of food doesn't 'match' the calorie content, so finds it harder to regulate the overall calories consumed. This may start to explain the emerging link between the consumption of diet drinks, obesity and increased risk of *metabolic syndrome*, characterised by hypertension, insulin resistance and high cholesterol.

So, we in western societies have access to plentiful, cheap, constantly available food that is so delicious that people find it hard to control their appetite. Manufacturers load food with sugar, fat and salt which encourages you to eat a lot of calories very quickly and prevents you from stopping, even when you're full. You can't rely on diet or healthy eating options as these may have high levels of artificial sweeteners that make it difficult for the brain to regulate calorie consumption.

At the same time that people are eating so much more, they are doing much less. People are less physically active than any previous generation and it is this, as well as the changes in eating habits, that upsets the balance between energy consumption and energy expenditure. The environment has changed so much that we hardly need to do any physical work. We have cars, washing machines, vacuum cleaners and lawn mowers to take the effort out of daily tasks and our entertainments, such as television and computer games, are often sedentary. The average person walks 189 miles a year, compared to 255 miles two decades ago, while time spent watching television has doubled since the 1960s.[8]

Social factors

Life events such as new relationships, divorce, illness, bereavement, a move of house, changes of work or financial situation, giving up smoking and even going on holiday can all affect your weight and make you vulnerable to weight gain. These events may influence your weight by making you less able to engage in healthy behaviours, such as loss of work meaning you have to give up gym membership; an accident forcing you to give up sports; or not having enough money to buy healthy food. Or they may make it easier to engage in unhealthy behaviours, such as having a fish and chip shop across the road; sharing a love of good food with your new partner; or comfort eating in response to distress.

Happy events and holidays

Many people are aware of the impact of stress and upset on their eating habits (this is discussed further below), but may not consider the impact of happier events. New relationships, marriage and holidays can all put you at risk of gaining weight.

Relationship contentment is frequently cited as a trigger for weight gain[9] and you may recognise a pattern of putting on weight when you are in a new relationship. This contentment weight may be the result of romantic meals out or takeaway pizzas in front of a video, less time to go to the gym, or feeling that you don't need to try quite so hard. Single people may work harder to manage their weight while they're dating and want to attract a partner. Research supports the view that the transition from single life to living with a partner increases the risk of weight gain.[10] One Australian study of 6,500 young women found that, over ten years, women with no partner and no baby gained on average 5kg; those with a partner and no baby gained almost 7kg; and if they had a partner and a baby they gained an average of 9kg.[11]

You may also recognise that you become less careful with your eating when on holiday and on special occasions. People on diets some-times find that a holiday triggers more uncontrolled eating that's hard to get back under control when the break is over. One study suggested that, rather than gaining weight steadily over the course of a year, people are most likely to put on weight at certain times, especially around Christmas. This study showed that people put on a relatively small amount, around half a kilogram, running up to Christmas but fail to lose the extra weight over the year so the weight accumulates. People who are already overweight are at risk of gaining more than this, an average of 2kg.[12]

Staying active

Most people understand that exercising and staying active is important in keeping weight under control. Exercise seems to be a key component in *maintaining* weight loss (that is, keeping the weight off once you've dieted successfully). Unfortunately, understanding the need to remain active is not the same as feeling motivated – overcoming the emotional, social and practical barriers to getting tired, sweaty and out of breath. You may have a job, children or parents to look after, the shopping and housework to do, and if you're lucky you may have some time left to relax with your friends or have a quiet evening in. The demands we now face are quite different from those of our ancestors. In the past people would be busy doing hard physical jobs and there were no washing machines or cars to make life easier. People didn't need to *think* about exercise, their lives provided them with more than enough activity. Physical activity is no longer a natural part of our lives, we have to plan and work at it. The time to exercise competes with time for other tasks; exercise is an excellent way of managing stress, but it may feel like finding time for exercise is a stress in itself.

It is clear that most people don't manage the level of exercise required to stay healthy. Current guidelines suggest that people need 150 minutes of moderate to vigorous exercise accumulated over the week in bouts of 10 minutes or more.[13] Moderate exercise doesn't necessarily mean going to the gym or the swimming pool, it can be any activity that leaves you slightly out of breath and a bit tired; a brisk walk, gardening or dancing can all count. Vigorous exercise, like cycling, running, aerobics or football, makes you breathe heavily and sweat. This level of physical activity is needed to reduce the risk of diabetes, colon cancer, breast cancer and cardiovascular disease, but it's estimated that only a third of adults reach these exercise goals with work commitments and lack of leisure time being the most common explanations.[14]

People who are overweight or obese are less likely to be managing this level of exercise and tend to spend more time doing sedentary (non-physical) activities. As well as the social pressures faced by us all – family commitments, long working hours, money worries – people who are overweight have additional challenges when it comes to taking regular exercise. Health and emotional barriers can be hard to overcome; self-consciousness, depression, low motivation, stress, fatigue, back and knee pain, and breathlessness can all make it difficult to maintain a routine of physical activity.

Sally had always struggled with her weight. With both children she'd put on quite a lot, but stayed as active as she could. She found that if she went to the gym two or three times a week and walked to the school every day she was able to keep her weight steady. Then, when she was 36, Sally had an accident in her car. She started to experience severe neck and back pain. She was not able to go to the gym – she could barely do the 15-minute walk to school! Sally felt hopeless about managing her weight and quickly gained a couple of stone. The frustration at not being able to do anything just made her want to eat more.

It can help to get support and encouragement for your exercise target. If you involve friends or family exercise can feel less of a chore. A cycle ride at the local park or a walk along the beach with others will be more fun and will increase your confidence. After weight loss surgery, keeping up a regular exercise programme is essential if you want the best possible results. See Chapter 8 for help planning a *realistic* and *sustainable* exercise programme. If you suffer from long-term back or joint pain that prevents you from exercising, you may want to speak to your GP about referral to a pain management programme that can support you with a gradual return to physical activity.

Giving up smoking

You probably know someone who has gained weight after they stopped smoking and started smoking again in order to get their weight back under control! On average people gain 4–5kg when they stop smoking, usually in the first six months. However, some smokers gain a lot more, up to 13kg, when they quit.[15] In general, the more cigarettes you smoked the more weight you're likely to gain.

There are a number of reasons you may gain weight when you give up smoking:

- Nicotine speeds up your resting metabolism, the energy required by the body to carry out its basic functions. When you smoke, your body burns calories at a faster rate and it's been estimated that smoking can cause you to burn an additional 200 calories a day.[16]
- Nicotine suppresses your appetite. It affects the part of your brain responsible for making you feel hungry. Increased appetite is one of the longest lasting effects of giving up cigarettes. Your sense of taste may also improve when you stop smoking, tempting you to eat more.
- Your food choices may change with an increased desire for sweet or high fat foods. Studies have shown that rats withdrawing from nicotine crave sugar.
- Food can act as a substitute for cigarettes as a way of dealing with boredom or stress. Comfort food may substitute for the relief you felt after smoking. Some people drink more alcohol when they quit smoking and this can also cause weight gain.
- Eating gives you something to do with your hands. Many ex-smokers find they miss the physical 'hand-to-mouth' habit of lighting and smoking a cigarette and snacking may replace this ritual.

Doctors have shown that, although ex-smokers tended to be 3–5kg heavier than current smokers, after five years there was no weight difference between ex-smokers and people who have never smoked, so it's worth persevering. Government advice is that the health gains from giving up smoking far outweigh the health risks associated with increased weight. The stress on your heart from smoking one packet of cigarettes a day is equivalent to being more than 40kg overweight![17]

Psychological factors: stress, emotion and eating

Controlled eating and failed diets

People who are severely overweight often have a long history of repeated attempts at dieting. You may have tried slimming clubs, liquid diets, high protein/low carbs, low GI, hypnotherapy, tablets that stop you absorbing fat, tablets that speed up your metabolism, tablets that make you urinate, healthy eating, calorie counting, soup diets and fruit diets.

People tend to see the main blocks to weight loss as being lack of energy or willpower; not having enough time; not having support from others for exercising; the high cost of healthy foods; and the greater pleasure in high fat foods.[18] However, despite the social, emotional and environmental barriers, many weight loss surgery patients do have a history of successful dieting, sometimes losing very substantial amounts of weight, and are well aware that their problem is with maintenance of weight loss. Anyone who has been on a diet, lost some weight then put it back on again will recognise how crushing this is and yet, it's the norm. You may feel you've been on a diet all your life and a sense of hopelessness in maintaining weight loss is a common reason for wanting bariatric surgery. Most dieters are aware of how hard it is to lose weight, and how easy it is to regain.

However much you tell yourself that *this time* it will be different, that you'll stick to the diet, keep up the exercise and never let yourself get big again, the reality is that most people regain weight lost through dieting. Almost inevitably the choices you face in our modern world are skewed towards weight gain over weight loss.[19] Biologically, dieting reduces fat stores (as you want it to) which in turn weakens the feedback signals that tell the brain that you have enough energy reserves. This diminished feedback leads to activation of the brain to stimulate hunger.[20] Subjective hunger and lowered levels of the 'full' neurohormones regulating appetite can persist for many months after a period of dieting, encouraging weight regain.[21] Repeated dieting and the yo-yoing of weight, known as weight cycling, can cause depression, increases the risk of uncontrolled eating[22] and may weaken immune function.[23]

Another effect of repeated dieting is that you become preoccupied with the foods you are not allowed to eat. You may actively try to restrict your eating and have certain foods that are 'forbidden' or 'bad'. People who consciously think about controlling their food intake are defined as 'restrained eaters', while people who eat on the basis of feeling hungry or full are termed 'unrestrained' or 'free' eaters. These terms do not refer to the *amount* of food you eat; both groups consume roughly the same number of calories each day.[24]

People who are overweight or obese are more likely to be restrained eaters, and it makes sense that people who know they are at risk of gaining weight actively control what they eat. However, it seems that the relationship between eating restraint and weight is more complicated; restrained eating appears to contribute to weight gain rather than protect against it. If you compare twins who have grown up together (thus controlling for environment and genetics) you still get an effect of restraint; the person showing more restrained eating is heavier than their twin, has a history of weight fluctuation and repeated diet attempts and is more likely to have gained weight recently.[25]

So, why does trying to control eating lead to weight gain? Studies show that people who show high levels of restraint are much more likely to overeat in response to stress compared to unrestrained eaters[26] while free eaters tend to lose their appetite. Perhaps restraint makes you more vulnerable to overeating in response to a whole range of situations when your control slips. Or possibly restraint increases the pleasure of food so when restraint is dropped the act of eating is more rewarding.[24]

We also know that restrained eaters who are very rigid in their food choices are more vulnerable to gaining weight than more flexible restrained eaters, so it may be strict food rules that cause problems. If you are trying to give up cigarettes, alcohol or drugs, any lapse is likely to be followed by a loss of control – this is known as the abstinence violation effect. If you are a strict dieter and you eat a *forbidden* food, you may overeat in response to this perceived loss of control.

Habitual eating

You may be aware of overeating, not because you are hungry or sad, but simply out of habit. Do you have a favourite chair for watching TV and do you ever snack while watching TV sitting in this chair? Over time you develop a conditioned response to a particular situation or setting. Even if you're not hungry – you may have just eaten a large meal – the conditioned response will make you think about eating as soon as you sit down. If you are a smoker or ex-smoker you may recognise this effect, experiencing a strong urge to smoke as soon as you have a drink placed in front of you in a pub. Working at the computer, going to the cinema and stopping at a petrol station are all common triggers for habitual eating.

You can make simple changes to help break these habits. You can decide only ever to eat at your kitchen table. You can change your furniture around so your favourite chair is facing a different angle (and then not snack when you're sitting in it). If you feel you must have a snack make yourself sit in the kitchen alone while you eat and the reduced stimulation will make eating less desirable.

Stress and emotional eating

> I was a comfort eater, if I was feeling emotional or fed up, I would eat, and then feel terribly guilty, which in turn makes you feel more miserable, so you eat more, it was a vicious circle.
>
> K, gastric bypass

Emotional eating, also known as comfort eating, is not uncommon; almost half of one American sample reported responding to stress by eating in order to feel better.[27] If you ask young women about their eating habits, many say they feel hungrier and make less healthy food choices when stressed, preferring chocolate, ice cream and fast foods. Conversely, people are more likely to eat healthy food when they feel good or if they've done some exercise.[28]

The relationship between weight gain and emotional factors is a complex one. Stress may lead to metabolic changes; it affects food choices, increasing preference for high fat, high sugar foods; it may mean you have less time for food preparation leading to a greater reliance on high calorie convenience food; and is likely to reduce physical activity.[29] All of these factors can result in an imbalance between energy consumption and expenditure.

The 'affect regulation model' suggests that some people comfort eat as a strategy to cope with painful emotions, such as anger, sadness or anxiety. Emotional eating may become more problematic if you have few other strategies for coping with difficult events or feelings or are less tolerant of emotional experience generally. Poor emotional regulation skills and difficulty in monitoring and modifying emotional reactions, have been linked with emotional problems and eating disorders.

According to affect regulation models[30] individuals who are feeling stressed, angry or distressed eat to comfort or calm themselves and to distract from the source of upset. Overeating is considered by some as a form of addictive behaviour[31] and being low or stressed can enhance the value of food, increasing food cravings and preoccupation with the thought of food. Being upset may also impact on people's ability to make a rational decision to resist food in favour of the long-term goal of weight loss. People who work hard to restrain their food intake, and those who eat emotionally, are most prone to this effect. So, emotional eaters seem to be hypersensitive to the rewarding qualities of food when they are in a negative mood, while non-emotional eaters tend to have less interest in food when upset.

So why does eating make you feel better (if only for a short time)? Stress occurs when you are faced with a threat. The stress is worse if the threat feels uncontrollable and it makes you feel frightened, and this includes the threat of social shame or failure. The purpose of the stress response is to prepare your body for 'fight or flight'. Various chemicals are released that ready the body for battle; blood flow is directed to the muscles and heart, and your breathing and heart rate become more rapid to supply oxygen to the muscles. Energy is directed away from the digestion of food and concern about reproduction, as these basic functions are less important at times of crisis. Because of this, animal studies usually show stress decreasing appetite and the urge to eat. However, animal studies have also shown that stress *increases* eating where there is access to highly palatable foods (that is, food high in fat and sugar)[32] and they are less likely to compensate for this extra stress eating by reduced food intake at other times.[33] While around a third of people decrease food intake and lose weight during stress, it is thought that the other two-thirds eat more.[34]

In the first chapter the major role that the hypothalamus plays in the regulation of appetite was discussed. The hypothalamus has been described as 'the drive centre of the brain, controlling hunger, thirst, lust, anger and arousal' (Brown 2000: 187).[35] It has a central role in coordinating the stress response, stimulating the release of cortisol, sometimes known as the 'stress hormone'. The greater the perceived threat the more cortisol is released. Cortisol increases hunger and reduces rational control of eating.[24] People who report more emotional eating may be more reactive, producing more cortisol when stressed. These people, like the animals in laboratory studies, eat more high fat food in response to experimental stress, which then blunts the stress response and reduces anxiety.

Both binge eaters and emotional eaters show high levels of cortisol and a greater urge to eat when faced with a stressful situation.[36,37] Binge eating represents a loss of control of eating behaviour and, like emotional eating, may also reflect problems in coping with difficult emotions. Binge eaters tend to experience negative emotions before a binge, which evaporates during the binge episode and then returns when the person has finished eating. After a binge episode you may feel upset or ashamed that you lost control of your eating. If you have frequent binge episodes and do not compensate for this by controlling food intake at other times, you are likely to experience weight gain. There's more information about binge eating in Chapter 5.

The release of stress chemicals has an impact on other systems that influence eating behaviour.[24] Stress chemicals promote the release of neuropeptide Y (NPY), which creates an urge to eat and reduces anxiety, and alters the brain reward system in ways that promote the hedonic (pleasure) value of food. They also activate the release of endogenous opioids (endorphins) which are designed to protect you from the ongoing negative effects of stress. These endorphins shut down the stress response, reduce pain and create a sense of well-being; they also increase eating of palatable foods. Raised cortisol may also increase insulin and leptin resistance so diminishing the strength of the body's *full* signals. In the modern world, we are faced much of the time with relatively minor, but repeated, stresses and this constant bombardment of daily hassles may be sufficient over time to disconnect appetite and eating behaviour from calorie need.

Childhood adversity

Given the link between emotions and eating behaviour, it's perhaps unsurprising that adult obesity has been linked to childhood adversity. Physical, sexual and emotional abuse as a child or the experience of domestic violence in the home significantly increases the risk of later obesity.[38] The more negative events the child is exposed to the more at risk they are of being obese as an adult.[39] Though extreme events have the strongest association with obesity, even general neglect or poor parental involvement all show some association with weight problems in later life. As well as being a risk factor for obesity, physical and emotional abuse during adolescence increases the risk of type 2 diabetes;[40] when girls in this study were five years old there was no difference in the body weight of girls reporting abuse compared to those that did not report abuse, but by their late teens the two groups were very different. By the time they were 30 there was a clear association between body mass index (BMI) and severity of childhood abuse, but even taking account of increased obesity the women who had been abused as children still showed greater risk of diabetes.

It is not fully understood why people who have had difficult experiences in childhood are vulnerable to becoming overweight or obese. It may be that the abuse makes you more likely to experience anxiety, depression or low self-esteem, affecting the ability to cope with difficult emotions and making people more likely to engage in emotional eating. Eating can become a means by which you *anaesthetise* your feelings; the act of putting food into your mouth and feeling your stomach becoming fuller can numb feelings of anger, sadness or emotional emptiness. It may be a strategy learnt as a young child, that eating makes you feel calmer and eases difficult thoughts and feelings. This kind of eating may be triggered by being alone or by feelings of abandonment.

Georgia was abused by her uncle from 9 to 14 years old. Her family didn't seem to see what was going on. Whenever she thought about telling someone, Georgia imagined how her mother would feel; she was scared the family would fall apart.

Instead of talking she began to eat. She would stay in her room where she kept a stash of crisps, chocolate and fizzy drinks. Sometimes she would eat so much that she'd feel sick, but while she was eating she forgot about what was happening. Eating and sleeping were the only things that gave Georgia a break. She'd look in the mirror and feel pleased that she'd soon be too big for him to push around.

Adults who were abused as children sometimes talk about their weight as protection from unwanted sexual attention; by becoming fatter you may feel psychologically distanced from your experience, or feel that being bigger makes you stronger and less desirable, and so less vulnerable.

If you have suffered from abuse or domestic violence and would like help and support there are organisations listed in the Resources section in Chapter 11. In Chapter 6 there are techniques you can practise to help cope with stress, upset and negative thoughts.

Biological factors: age, illness and genetics

Age

Studies have shown that people are getting fatter earlier in their lives and staying fat for longer.[41] The majority of overweight adults were overweight by five years old[42] and children with poor exercise and eating habits are very likely to become adults with poor eating and exercise habits[43] so around three-quarters of severely overweight adolescents will go on to be obese adults.[44]

Obesity is becoming a major health issue for children; around three in ten children between 2 and 15 years old are significantly overweight.[45] Half of these are already classified as obese, which means their weight is likely to be having a negative impact on their health. Even more worrying is the fact that around a fifth of three to five-year-olds in the UK are overweight or obese.[46]

These children are faced with the same challenges and difficulties as adults in managing their weight. They have access to the same range of high fat, high sugar foods and the joys of sedentary distractions in the form of television, computer games and social networking sites. Some children are becoming so overweight it is affecting their health and quality of life. They are at risk of developing type 2 diabetes and hypertension as teenagers[47] and are vulnerable to sleep apnoea, heart disease and premature death as they enter early adulthood.[48]

Around 20 per cent of children face an overweight adolescence and the psychological consequences of this can be profound. Obese teenagers are vulnerable to depression, disabling self-consciousness, low self-esteem[49] and even suicidal behaviour.[50] Negative feelings about themselves, and unkind comments from others, take a toll on social confidence and body image. Being overweight or obese at school puts children at heightened risk of being bullied, which in turn affects

---

'I'm not overweight, everyone I know looks like me . . .'

Over the years, people's perceptions of what is overweight has shifted upwards[51] and our social network can have a powerful influence on our weight. Our risk of becoming obese is increased by 57 per cent if a friend becomes obese, by 40 per cent if a sibling becomes obese, and by 37 per cent if a spouse or partner becomes obese.[52]

Children who have overweight parents are more likely to be overweight. In part this will be due to our genetic inheritance and we learn how and what to eat from the people around us. But there is also another way in which family and friends influence children's weight. A study has shown that young people who are overweight are more likely to misjudge their weight compared to a normal weight kid if they have obese parents or friends. In other words, children who are overweight judge themselves as weighing less than they really do, because they have got used to seeing other overweight people. As their excess weight is 'normalised' by the people around them, these young people may be less motivated to make changes to their diet or exercise in order to lose weight.[53]

---

educational achievement, social development and emotional well-being. A lack of opportunity for social success may force the young person into a smaller and smaller 'comfort zone', spending time in their room with only the television, computer and food for company.[54]

> I put weight on when I hit puberty. I would eat and eat, but feel really bad about it. I was bullied because I was fat and I would make myself sick to get rid of the food that I had eaten, but because I hated being sick I stopped fairly quickly.
>
> K, gastric bypass

If you are worried about your child's weight, you can speak to your GP or school nurse who will assess your child's overall health and support you in establishing a healthy eating and activity plan with your child. They can also refer your child to MEND (Mind, Exercise, Nutrition . . . Do it!) who organise healthy lifestyle programmes for children and families.

As we get older there is a tendency for people to put on weight, possibly due to decreased activity and changes in metabolic rate due to lowered muscle mass. For women in particular, there are certain times in life when there is an increased risk of gaining weight. Pregnancy is a risk point for weight gain, with more than a third of women showing excessive weight increase[55] putting them at greater risk of caesarean section and poor post-pregnancy weight loss.[56] Gaining excess weight during pregnancy may trigger a subsequent loss of control over weight and lead to continued weight gain after pregnancy.

Later in life, the menopause (when a woman stops having periods) is a time when you are again at risk of gaining weight. Post-menopausal women are vulnerable to gaining weight (on average around 3kg) due to lowered resting metabolic rate and decreased physical activity.[57] There is a change in body shape, with more fat settling around the abdomen, and a decrease in lean body mass which lowers resting metabolism. This post-menopausal weight gain carries a greater risk of cardiovascular disease, diabetes, high blood pressure, arthritis and hormone-dependent breast and endometrial (lining of the uterus) cancers.

Health and medication

Poor health or disability is one of the most common biological factors that affect weight, primarily because it makes you less able to be active. There are, however, certain conditions that have a direct effect on weight.

Cushing's syndrome

Cushing's syndrome (sometimes called hyperadrenocorticism or hyper-corticism) is caused by high levels of cortisol in the blood, due to the growth of a tumour on the adrenal or pituitary glands or treatment with corticosteriods. Cushing's disease can result in rapid weight gain, especially on the face and around the waist. Other symptoms can include high blood pressure; excessive sweating; dark-coloured stretch marks on the stomach; painful joints; sleeplessness; facial hair; reduced sex drive; depression and anxiety. If untreated, Cushing's syndrome makes people vulnerable to the development of type 2 diabetes, osteoporosis and heart disease.

Hypothyroidism

The thyroid gland is a small gland sitting underneath the Adam's apple at the front of the neck. It produces the hormone, thyroxine, that helps control your metabolic rate. In hypothyroidism, the thyroid gland doesn't make enough thyroxine, the metabolic rate slows down, you burn fewer calories and are likely to gain weight. Some women develop hypothyroidism after having a baby (known as *postpartum thyroiditis*). Symptoms include loss of muscle tone; tiredness; increased sensitivity to cold; joint pain; muscle cramp; depression; carpal tunnel syndrome; thinning hair; osteoporosis; itchy skin; changes in the menstrual cycle; and irritability. Less commonly people with hypothyroidism can experience problems with memory and concentration.

Polycystic ovary syndrome (PCOS)[58]

PCOS affects around 10 per cent of women and is a major cause of infertility. It is caused by small cysts (like little blisters) growing in the ovaries which disrupt the balance of hormones, and makes it less likely that you will ovulate. It is associated with weight gain, especially around the abdomen, irregular periods, acne and facial hair. Women with PCOS are at greater risk of type 2 diabetes, high blood pressure, dyslipidaemia, cardiovascular disease and miscarriage. Management of PCOS is a low calorie, low carbohydrate diet combined with regular exercise and some medications may help.

Insulinoma[59]

Insulinoma is a rare condition (there are only two to three new cases per million people a year) caused by a benign tumour on the pancreas that produces extra insulin. The excess insulin lowers blood sugar levels, causing you to feel hungry and wanting to eat more and it can be associated with rapid weight gain. You may also experience head-aches, fatigue, confusion and blurred vision. Treatment is through surgical removal of the tumour.

Your GP will have checked for all likely medical reasons for your weight gain before referring you for weight loss surgery. When you are assessed for weight loss surgery you may see an *endocrinologist* (a doctor specialised in the diagnosis and treatment of conditions affecting hormones) who will complete a thorough assessment of any underlying medical problems. There is more information about this in Chapter 5.

Serious illnesses like insulinoma are fortunately rare and even the more common disorders, such as PCOS or Cushing's syndrome, only affect a small proportion of the population. Many more people are affected by the side effects of medication taken for other medical conditions. Medication is a major factor in many people's battle with weight and a number of prescription drugs are associated with weight gain, though the effects vary from person to person.

There are a number of ways in which prescription medication can cause you to gain weight:

• A prescription drug may increase appetite or cause you to crave certain foods. Insulin, used in the management of diabetes, is known to cause weight gain, probably due to the episodes of hypoglycaemia (low blood sugar) which stimulate appetite.

- Some drugs affect metabolism, causing the body to burn calories more slowly or to store fat. Corticosteroids make the body less able to absorb blood glucose, leading to fat deposits around the tummy. Some antidepressants seem to reduce appetite, but still result in weight gain as a result of changes to resting metabolism.
- Some drugs are likely to make you less active (e.g. beta blockers for high blood pressure) as they cause fatigue.
- Medication for bipolar disorder and some anti-depressants give you a dry mouth, causing you to drink more. If you drink high calorie drinks this can cause weight gain.

A number of drugs prescribed by psychiatrists for depression (SSRIs and tricyclic antidepressants), bipolar disorder (lithium), and psychotic disorders (especially the 'atypical' antipsychotics such as olanzepine and clozapine) can cause weight gain.[60] It is thought these psychiatric medicines affect the leptin system (the satiety hormone) and the hypothalamus; they can cause increased appetite for sweet foods and carbohydrate cravings; and may affect resting metabolic rate. It's important to recognise that you might also have weight gain as a direct result of the symptoms of depression; lowered motivation means you are generally less active, you may sleep longer and engage in more emotional eating.

With all medications, your doctor should give you information about whether it makes you vulnerable to gaining weight and offer advice about how to manage this. Patients sometimes become so distressed about weight gain that they stop taking their medication. This can have a serious effect on health and may result in a deterioration or relapse in the condition. You should not stop taking a medication that you think is making you gain weight without speaking to your doctor. The effects of discontinuing medication may be far more serious than the increase in weight. Your GP should monitor weight gain and if necessary offer an alternative medication.

The genetics of obesity

You heard earlier about the sheer pace of the obesity epidemic; in just the last 20 years the western world has seen an immense increase in the numbers of people affected. Because of the speed of this change, many people have dismissed genetic factors as having an insignificant role in obesity, arguing that there could not have been any important changes in the genetic makeup of the population in such a short time. However, it now seems likely that genetic variations interact with the modern environment to make some people susceptible to gaining weight.

Genes are present in all of your cells. They hold information about how to run the body, like an incredibly complex instruction manual. Genes are passed to you from your parents; you have 23 pairs of chromosomes, one set from your mother and one from your father. Your genes determine the colour of your eyes, your height, the shape of your nose and the million other variations in physique and temperament that make up who you are. Studies of identical twins and adopted children suggest that genetic factors contribute 45–75 per cent of variation in weight.[61]

Variations in genes reflect adaption to your environment over many hundreds of thousands of years. People living in places where they faced famine would have been more likely to survive (and therefore have children and pass on their genes) if they were efficient at storing fat to see them through hard times. Their descendants are said to have a 'thrifty phenotype'; their bodies maintain efficient metabolism which allows excess calories to be put into fat storage. Faced with a modern environment, with endless supplies of high energy food, the body still acts as if there's a risk of famine and continues to store fat.[62]

The first major discovery in the genetics of obesity was the *OB* mouse. This poor mouse was the result of a spontaneous genetic mutation. He wanted to eat too much, had a low metabolism and got very fat. By breeding from this mouse, scientists could identify the source of the problem and called it the OB gene. They showed that this gene is responsible for telling fat cells to produce leptin, the hormone that tells you when you have got enough energy stored in fat cells. Since then rare cases of severe obesity in humans have been shown to be the result of a lack of leptin due to the OB gene mutation and, for these people, treatment with leptin can produce remarkable weight loss.[63] The OB gene is an example of a *monogenic* condition – it's caused by a problem with just a single gene. Most obese people have a normal OB gene and treatment with leptin has no affect on their weight, but geneticists have discovered other monogenic conditions linked with obesity in humans, including variations in the MC4R receptor gene[64] linked to binge eating[65] and the FTO gene[66] which is associated with difficulty controlling eating, higher consumption of fat and decreased satiety.[62] Other gene mutations seem to protect against excessive weight gain.[67]

While rare genetic or chromosomal abnormalities can produce extreme obesity syndromes, in most cases genetic vulnerability to obesity is due to the influence of a number of genes (*polygenic*). Where specific mutations in certain genes produce severe childhood obesity, small variations in these same genes seem to predispose individuals to being overweight. Vulnerability to obesity is likely to be the result of complex interactions between genes and the environment that affect appetite regulation, eating behaviour[68] and the proportion of fat to lean body tissue. To date around 130 different genes influencing obesity have been discovered, including genes that affect the chemical signalling of hunger and satiety, energy expenditure and the growth of fat cells.[69] By exploring the biological causes of obesity, genetic research is helping to reduce the stigma of obesity; it will continue to offer insight into the mechanisms underlying appetite and energy balance and offers hope in the development of dietary programmes or medication to manage or prevent obesity.

> We must think of human food intake not as an entirely voluntarily controllable phenomenon but one driven by powerful biological signals from relatively primitive brain areas.
>
> Farooqi and O'Rahilly 2007: 38[61]

Your weight journey

This chapter has covered the environmental, social, psychological and biological factors that can make you vulnerable to gaining weight and you may recognise some of these influences in yourself. It is hoped you will understand a little more about your weight journey and perhaps can be less critical of your own battle with weight as you reflect on the various influences that have contributed to your difficulties.

When you meet the dietitian for your assessment before surgery, he/she will be interested in knowing whether you are able to understand and reflect on the factors that have influenced your weight gain. You can use this exercise to help create a picture of your weight journey – a map of the changes in your weight and the events that have affected these changes over the years. It may be helpful to use this map to think about your response to stress or unhappiness, the impact of relationships on your eating habits, circumstances that enabled you to lose weight successfully, and your feelings about your weight and appearance.

Mapping your weight journey

Figure 2.2 is an illustration of a weight journey. On a large piece of paper, draw a line horizontally across the centre of the page. On the left end of the line, write the year you were born. On the other end, write the current year. Fill in your age between the two dates along the line (e.g. 10, 20, 30 years, etc.). Above the line mark on the weight you were at different ages. It doesn't matter if you use stones or kilograms, or you could use your clothes size if you can't remember your weight. Try to build up a detailed picture of how your weight has changed over the years. Use these weights to draw a line showing the ups and downs in your weight.

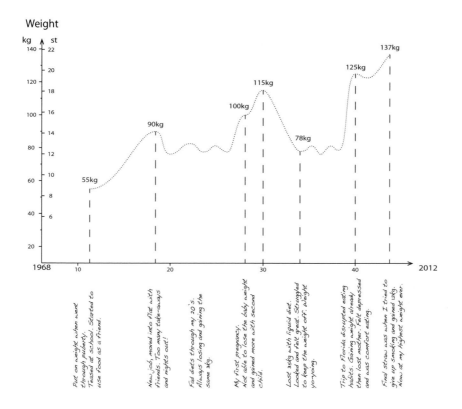

Figure 2.2 A weight journey

When you have a clear idea of your weight line, write down important events in your life below the centre line. These may be happy experiences (a great holiday, having your first child) or less happy (being bullied at school, losing a parent). Again try to build up a full picture of the important events in your life. You may want to ask other people (your husband, parents, best friend) what they can recall, but remember that what's been important for you may not be the same as for other people – it's your experience that counts.

You should now have a map that shows the changes in your weight and life events that occurred around the same time. Use this map to think about the following questions. You may want to write down your thoughts on the back of the paper.

- Have times of weight gain been associated with particular life events? Have the life events tended to be happy, sad or both?
- Do I eat in response to stress and upset?
- How have my activity/exercise levels changed over the years?

- Have the people in my life (parents, partners, friends) affected my eating? Has their influence been helpful or unhelpful?
- Have I gained weight in response to being left alone or bereaved?
- At what time was my weight most stable? What helped me keep my weight steady?
- When have I been most successful in losing weight? What was going on in my life then?

The more you understand the influences on your eating behaviour and weight, the better prepared you will be to make the changes required by weight loss surgery. Your past experience can give you a good idea about high risk situations in the future as well as allowing you to recognise what has helped you keep your weight stable in the past. If your weight journey suggests high levels of emotional eating (with weight gain at times of high stress or upset), it may be important to resolve this issue and develop alternative strategies for coping with distress before proceeding with surgery. See Chapter 6 for information on useful distress management techniques.

3

'I just want a normal life':
the impact of obesity

While some people who are very overweight do not suffer in terms of their health or emotional well-being, most people who look to weight loss surgery do so because their health has deteriorated to the extent that they no longer have a good quality of life or because they feel low and isolated because of their weight and appearance.

This chapter covers some of the main physical and emotional difficulties faced by people who are obese. When you are being assessed for weight loss surgery, these health problems, called *comorbidities*, will be considered and may affect your eligibility for surgery.

Physical health

> [Before surgery I had] heart failure, high blood pressure, sleep apnoea, exhaustion, constant pain in feet, ankles and hips [and] pain in my back and neck.
>
> J, sleeve gastrectomy

It is no longer possible to view body fat as inert tissue, storing energy but having no relationship or interaction with the rest of the body. Fat acts as a dynamic organ and, when at healthy levels, has an important role in protecting bones and organs, regulating hormones, the immune system and women's reproductive function. When people have high levels of body fat it can unbalance other systems, causing damage to blood vessels and fostering insulin resistance.

Studies have shown that obesity affects more people and has a greater impact on chronic health problems and the cost of health care than smoking, heavy drinking and poverty. These researchers described the impact of obesity as 'like aging from 30 to 50 [years]' in terms of long-term health conditions.[1,2]

Being overweight is associated with a greatly increased risk of type 2 diabetes, coronary heart disease, stroke, hypertension, gall bladder disease, insulin resistance, non-alcoholic fatty liver, sleep apnoea, asthma, breathlessness, daytime sleepiness, osteoarthritis and dyslipidaemia. Over two-thirds of weight loss surgery patients with a body mass index (BMI) of more than 50 have three or more comorbid conditions.[3]

The National Institute for Health and Clinical Excellence (NICE) outlined the risk of developing health problems if you are overweight or obese compared to a normal weight person (Table 3.1).

Diabetes

Diabetes (also known as diabetes mellitus) is a chronic condition characterised by having too much sugar in the blood. The amount of blood sugar is controlled by insulin, a hormone produced by the pancreas. Insulin allows sugar to be taken into cells and converted into energy or stored for future use.

There are two types of diabetes; type 1, where the pancreas makes little or no insulin, and type 2 where the body has become resistant to insulin and the pancreas can no longer keep up with demand. Type 2 diabetes is by far the most common form of diabetes, usually starting in adulthood, and is closely linked with excess weight. Symptoms can include tiredness, excessive thirst and blurred vision. Type 2 diabetes can sometimes be managed by following a healthy lifestyle initially, but the ability of the body to make insulin decreases over time ultimately requiring medication or insulin injections.

Table 3.1 Health problems related to obesity[4]

Level of increased risk	Health problems due to the metabolic effect of obesity	Health problems due to the physical effect of obesity
Greatly increased risk	Type 2 diabetes	Sleep apnoea
	Gall bladder disease	Breathlessness
	Hypertension	Asthma
	Dyslipidaemia	Social isolation
	Insulin resistance	Depression
	Non-alcoholic fatty liver	Daytime sleepiness
Moderately increased risk	Coronary heart disease	Osteoarthritis
	Stroke	Respiratory disease
	Gout	Hernia
Slightly increased risk	Cancer	Varicose veins
	Impaired fertility	Musculoskeletal problems
	Polycystic ovaries	Back pain
	Skin problems	Stress incontinence
	Cataracts	Oedema/cellulitis

Diabetes can lead to grave medical problems, including blindness and limb amputation, and being overweight or obese increases the likelihood of serious complications in people with diabetes.[5] Diabetes also significantly increases your risk of developing coronary heart disease even if your blood sugar levels are well controlled.[6] Almost a third of weight loss surgery patients in the UK have type 2 diabetes.[3]

Cardiovascular disease[7]

Cardiovascular disease refers to diseases that affect the heart and blood vessels and includes coronary heart disease and stroke. Coronary heart disease is the cause of death for one in four men and one in six women. It is caused by the build-up of fatty deposits (*atherosclerosis*) in the arteries supplying oxygen to the heart muscles. This restricts the blood supply to the heart causing pain (*angina*) and, if the arteries become completely blocked, a heart attack (*myocardial infarction*).

> [I had surgery] to avoid having heart surgery, my cardiologist informed me that 90 per cent of my heart problems were due to my excess weight.
>
> J, sleeve gastrectomy

The risk of coronary heart disease is greatly increased by being overweight or obese, smoking, having high blood pressure, high cholesterol and a sedentary (inactive) lifestyle. Obesity raises the risk because it is linked to diabetes, high blood pressure, raised levels of 'bad' cholesterol and lower levels of helpful cholesterol.

A stroke occurs if an artery supplying the brain becomes blocked, or an artery bleeds into the brain, cutting off the oxygen supply. Sometimes the blockage is temporary, causing a *transient ischaemic attack* (TIA) or *mini-stroke*.

Hypertension[7]

Blood pressure refers to the pressure of the blood as it travels through the arteries. When your blood pressure is taken you are given two numbers; the first number is the highest level of pressure that is reached when your heart pumps blood into the arteries (*systolic blood pressure*). The second number (*diastolic blood pressure*) is the lowest pressure reached as the heart relaxes between beats. A healthy blood pressure is below 140/85. Hypertension is diagnosed when your blood pressure is consistently higher than 140/90. It does not usually cause any symptoms, but it means that the heart has to work harder, causing the heart muscles to thicken and the walls of the arteries to become weaker. As well as increased risk of heart attack, hypertension also makes you more vulnerable to strokes, kidney failure and congestive heart failure. Almost half of very overweight adults have high blood pressure.[8]

Dyslipidaemia[7]

Dyslipidaemia is the medical term for high levels of certain fats (*lipids*), called cholesterol and triglycerides, in the blood.

There are two types of cholesterol:

- High density lipoprotein (HDL) cholesterol – sometimes called *good* cholesterol.
- Low-density lipoprotein (LDL) cholesterol – sometimes called *bad* cholesterol.

Too much LDL cholesterol in the blood increases *atherosclerosis* – the build-up of fatty deposits in the arteries – and so increases your risk of heart disease, stroke and high blood pressure. *Good* HDL cholesterol, on the other hand, seems to clean up excess cholesterol from the blood and protects against atherosclerosis. People are particularly at risk if they have high levels of LDL and low levels of HDL cholesterol.

Triglycerides[6] are fats present in the blood which, together with cholesterol, form the blood lipids. They come from the fat eaten in foods, such as meat and dairy products, and are also made by the body from other sources of energy, like carbohydrates. Calories from a meal

---

What is metabolic syndrome?[9]

Metabolic syndrome is a loss of metabolic balance in the body due to excess weight. It is diagnosed when a person has at least three of the following conditions:

- A high waist measurement (over 35 inches for women, 40 inches for men).
- Elevated blood sugar levels (diabetes or insulin resistance).
- High blood pressure.
- High triglyceride levels.
- Low levels of *good* cholesterol.

Metabolic syndrome increases the risk of coronary heart disease and stroke. It is estimated that around 25 per cent of American adults have metabolic syndrome.[10]

that are not used to produce energy are converted to triglycerides and transported to fat cells to be stored. Like LDL cholesterol, high levels of triglycerides in the blood increase the risk of coronary heart disease. Around a fifth of weight loss surgery patients have dyslipidaemia.[3]

Obstructive sleep apnoea (OSA)

Sleep apnoea is caused by obstruction of the airway. It is characterised by pauses in breathing (apnoea means *without breath*) which occur repeatedly throughout the night. The main signs of sleep apnoea are snoring and daytime sleepiness. It is often the patient's partner that notices that they stop breathing for short periods of time. Almost half of patients assessed for weight loss surgery have moderate or severe sleep apnoea.[11]

OSA is managed through the use of a CPAP (short for *continuous positive airway pressure*) machine, a mask that pushes air into the lungs to prevent any interruptions to breathing, or the variable pressure (VPAP).

Closely linked to OSA is a problem called *obesity hypoventilation syndrome* in which very overweight people fail to breathe rapidly or deeply enough to get an adequate oxygen supply, leading to high carbon dioxide (CO_2) levels in the blood. This puts strain on the heart and may result in symptoms of heart failure, such as fatigue, breathlessness, palpitations and swollen legs. Extreme overweight is also associated with adult-onset asthma severe enough to restrict daily activities.[12]

Arthritis

Obesity is closely linked to the development of painful osteoarthritis of the knee and hip[13] which impacts on mobility and restricts everyday activities. Bariatric patients often also experience chronic back, foot and ankle pain that interferes with their ability to work,[14] socialise, exercise and engage in leisure activities. Because of rising obesity, the rate of disability in younger adults is increasing rapidly; there has been a 50 per cent increase in 30- and 40-year-olds who are restricted in their ability to care for themselves or carry out day-to-day tasks.[15]

> Chronic arthritis and fibromyalgia [made it] very hard to walk because of severe pain.
>
> J, gastric bypass

Cancer[16]

Obesity is known to significantly increase the risk of many kinds of cancer including breast, bowel, uterine and oesophageal cancer and a number of less common types of cancer. It is the most important avoidable cause of cancer after smoking. It is estimated that up to 15 per cent of cases of post-menopause breast cancer, 15 per cent of cases of bowel cancer, 35 per cent cases of oesophageal adenocarcinoma and 50 per cent of cases of uterine cancer are caused by excessive weight.

Non-alcoholic fatty liver disease

Non-alcoholic fatty liver disease (*NAFLD*) occurs when excess fat is deposited in the liver (not due to excessive consumption of alcohol) and is linked to insulin resistance and metabolic syndrome.[17] People with NAFLD don't usually have any symptoms, though they sometimes report tiredness or dull abdominal discomfort, and it's generally only identified during routine blood tests. NAFLD can cause inflammation in the liver, a more serious condition with an increased risk of cirrhosis.

Fertility and pregnancy

Women who are severely overweight are more prone to fertility problems. Polycystic ovary syndrome[5] (PCOS) is a hormonal disorder causing irregular periods, infertility, weight gain and excess hair on the face and body. It is a common condition, affecting up to 10 per cent of adult women. It has been estimated that 15 per cent of women seeking weight loss surgery have a diagnosis of PCOS and fertility problems are often a motivation for wanting surgery.[18]

> My main reason [for wanting weight loss surgery] was that my husband and I have been trying for a baby for three years. We had had every test and nothing is wrong with either of us. Our fertility consultant told me that it is because I am obese, and all the time I am so fat we will never fall naturally.
>
> K, gastric bypass

Obesity also causes women to encounter more difficulties during pregnancy and childbirth, including gestational hypertension, pre-eclampsia, pregnancy-onset diabetes, spontaneous miscarriage, need for emergency caesarean section, maternal death and stillbirth.[19,20,21]

Gastro-oesophageal reflux disease (GORD)

Reflux disease is the result of acid from the stomach coming up into the oesophagus (the tube that runs from the mouth to the stomach), causing inflammation of the oesophagus and ongoing symptoms of heartburn or difficulty swallowing.

Stress incontinence

Obesity is a significant risk factor for stress incontinence for women[22] due to increased intra-abdominal pressure, which puts strain on the pelvic floor. Obesity may also affect the neurological and muscular function of the urinary system.[23]

Life expectancy

As obesity puts people at much greater risk of these health problems, it is perhaps unsurprising that it reduces life expectancy. It is thought that in England alone, more than 30,000 deaths are due to obesity.[24] The risk of death through cardiovascular disease, cancer and 'all causes' increases not simply with degree of obesity, but also with how long a person has been obese.[25] To put it in context, a 25-year-old obese man has a 22 per cent reduction in expected lifespan – the loss of 12 years of life.[26]

Impact of obesity on emotional health and quality of life

Obesity clearly affects people's health-related quality of life, through the impact of physical ill-health and the social or work limitations they cause. The more overweight a person is the greater the limitations they face[27] and simple daily tasks become difficult; walking, climbing stairs, dressing and personal care, rather than being carried out without thought, feel burdensome. Almost three-quarters of bariatric patients are unable to climb three flights of stairs without a rest.[3]

Severe overweight prevents or restricts people's ability to take part in activities they enjoy, be it going to the theatre or taking their children to the park. Physical limitations, and the distress and frustration they cause, are often a major motivator for people seeking weight loss surgery. Patients are often unable to work or socialise because of their physical limitations or fear of negative reactions from others. Poor physical quality of life, reduced life choices and social isolation, increase the risk of distress and anxiety.

Obesity and emotional well-being

Severely overweight people are more likely to have experienced depression, other mood disorders and anxiety.[28] Two-thirds of weight loss surgery patients have a history of emotional problems and around 40 per cent have a current mental health difficulty.[29] The symptoms of depression are low mood, tearfulness, irritability, poor motivation and loss of interest, reduced concentration, feeling hopeless about the future and self-critical, and possibly suicidal thoughts. The impact of obesity on emotional health is so profound that people with a BMI over 50 have a 120 per cent increased risk of attempted suicide compared to people with normal-range BMI.[30]

It is known that weight problems can both cause, and be caused by, depression. So obese people (particularly women and people who are severely obese) have a 55 per cent increased risk of developing depression, and a depressed person has a similarly increased risk of becoming obese. It is likely that depression makes people vulnerable to gaining weight due to unhealthy lifestyles, lowered motivation to diet, emotional eating and the effect of medication. Conversely, obesity causes depression through the impact of various psychosocial factors, including body dissatisfaction, social stigma, lowered self-esteem and social confidence, chronic pain and the physical restrictions that come with weight.[31]

Many very overweight people are highly conscious of the potential for negative reactions from others, feel inhibited from going out socially and are vulnerable to developing generalised anxiety, social phobia and panic attacks.[28] For some this anxiety is so great that they become withdrawn from all social activities.

Millie described herself as low and lonely; she pretends to be cheerful, but feels ostracised by others because of her appearance. She has stopped going out and avoids her friends. Sometimes life feels so difficult that she wishes she just wouldn't wake up in the morning. She would never harm herself, but she feels so alone.

There are mixed findings about the impact of emotional problems on outcome with weight loss surgery, and most research studies show that people with depression or anxiety do well. However people with severe and long-standing mental health problems sometimes experience poor weight loss and a worsening of their emotional state after surgery. If you are experiencing severe depression or anxiety you may need additional support before or after weight loss surgery. There is information about how you can access psychological therapy in Chapter 11.

Body image distress

People who seek weight loss surgery often feel deeply unhappy with their appearance. They may feel disgusted by their own body and believe that everyone around them feels equally repulsed. They speak about how the weight doesn't feel like 'them' – that they are trapped inside a false body from which they can't escape. They may seek to make themselves invisible, covering themselves with baggy clothes or simply never go out, too afraid of comments as they walk down the street.

Stunkard and Mendelson (1967)[32] described a pattern of body image disparagement in some obese people, characterised by a preoccupation with negative thoughts about their body, feeling it to be ugly and contemptible, and a belief that others view them with hostility. This distress affects people's ability to work and socialise and they are more likely to suffer symptoms of depression.[33] The negative impact on self-esteem and body image is greatest in very overweight people who have internalised anti-fat attitudes and stereotypes.[34]

Weight discrimination and stigma

> The year before I had surgery, I applied for 1,000 jobs when I was made redundant and had close to 150 interviews where they were all very excited by me. But I never had an offer . . . wonder why? Because my looks let me down I'm sure. I find this disgusting and terrible, but it is out there and it happens.
>
> A, gastric bypass

The pervasive discrimination shown against obese people has been described as the *last safe prejudice*.[35] In one study 80 per cent of pre-surgery bariatric patients felt they *always* or *usually* experienced discrimination from others because of their weight.[36]

Obese people have been shown to suffer discrimination and stigma in all areas of their life, from housing and education through to work opportunities and relationships.[37] Severely overweight adolescents face bullying, social isolation[38] and are less likely to achieve academically.[39] Obese adults are less likely to be offered a job, are more likely to be viewed as lazy or unreliable in the workplace, are offered fewer promotions and tend to earn less than normal weight colleagues.[40] They are more likely to be long-term unemployed and have a lower family income.[41]

Stigma has been described as a *mark* that links undesirable characteristics.[42] The more a disease is seen as being under the person's control the more stigmatising it is and the more social rejection people face.[43] Obesity is broadly viewed by the public as being highly under personal control, representing a failure of willpower. Rather than addressing the environmental conditions that cause obesity, our society blames the victim and perpetuates the view that obesity is the 'mark of a defective person'.[44]

People's *failure* to conform to social norms to be slim, active and fit is perceived as evidence of a flawed character, leading to *shaming* strategies to pressurise people to conform.[45] In reality, the experience of weight stigma tends to make people eat *less* healthily and feel *less* able to exercise.[46,47] Rather than motivating or encouraging people to manage their weight we know that negative responses from others can lead to disordered eating such as binge episodes[48] and depression.[49]

> I was never that ashamed of being large and often have fought against discrimination, because we are not all the same and should not be expected to be so, and if you feel happy and healthy why should we have to conform.
>
> A, gastric bypass

Vicious cycle of excessive weight, low mood and poor quality of life

We have seen is this chapter the impact of obesity on your physical health, emotional well-being, life opportunities and quality of life. These factors interact with each other, restricting the physical, economic and psychological resources people can access to deal with the problem, as illustrated in Figure 3.1.

It is this vicious trap that bariatric loss surgery seeks to reverse. With the weight loss produced by surgery, people often experience improvements in health, mood and confidence and so feel more able to make changes to their life, becoming more active and social. For some, weight loss surgery offers everything that they hoped for, but for others the path is less smooth and they encounter challenges and obstacles that make the journey to their desired life seem just as far away. We will be looking at these differing outcomes in later chapters.

Summary

Severe overweight is associated with a range of health problems, including diabetes, coronary heart disease, high blood pressure, sleep apnoea, breathing difficulties, arthritis and cancer. These disorders are termed *comorbidities* and will be considered during your assessment for surgery. Over two-thirds of weight loss surgery patients with a BMI over 50 have three or more comorbid conditions. These health problems reduce life expectancy, restrict day-to-day activities and have a profound impact on quality of life. Simple tasks like climbing stairs and personal care can become major challenges.

Obese people are often unable to work or socialise because of their physical limitations or fear of negative reactions from other and are vulnerable to experiencing feelings of depression and anxiety. Obesity can lead to depression due to lowered self-esteem and social confidence, body dissatisfaction, social stigma and discrimination.

Obesity is broadly viewed by the public as being under personal control, representing a lack of willpower. Rather than addressing the environmental conditions that cause obesity, our society blames the

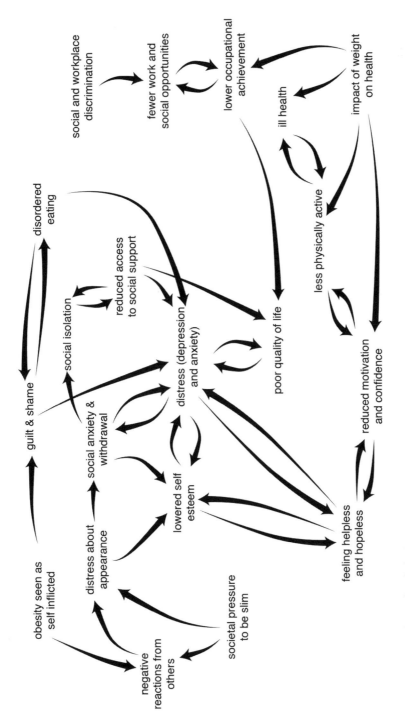

Figure 3.1 Negative cycle of obesity

victim and perpetuates the view that obesity is the result of personal failure and weakness. The pervasive discrimination shown against obese people has been described as the 'last safe prejudice' and is evident in the discrimination severely overweight people face in education, employment opportunities, earning power and healthcare.

Weight loss surgery seeks to reverse the vicious cycle of poor health, reduced opportunities, social discrimination, low self-esteem and diminished emotional well-being and quality of life. For many people surgery has a profoundly positive impact on their life, offering improvements in physical and emotional health. The next chapter will look at how to access weight loss surgery, find out whether you fit the criteria for surgery and consider your personal readiness for taking on the dramatic changes to your relationship with food and alterations to your lifestyle required for a successful outcome.

4

Accessing weight loss surgery

[My advice is] research well; choose a good bariatric team; stay within the UK; read about the changes you'll need to make and prepare for them; join a support group before surgery.

C, gastric bypass

The decision to have weight loss surgery is never going to be easy and you want to be sure that you will get the best possible care. In the UK the choice is between looking for funding through the NHS or paying privately. These routes both have benefits and disadvantages. Clearly the primary benefit of NHS surgery is that it is free and you can be confident that you will receive comprehensive follow-up care, but you will face strict rules about who is eligible for funding and there may be a long waiting time. Going privately offers a shorter wait and you may be able to have surgery at a hospital nearer home, and at a time that suits you, however the cost can be prohibitive and private clinics are variable in the quality of follow-up care included in the package.

Weight loss surgery with the NHS

I spoke to my GP and explained that I wanted to do something about my weight . . . I had tried slimming tablets and attended weight management classes. They organised a full set of blood tests, did my blood pressure and weighed me . . . She said once the results were back she would write recommending I had weight loss surgery.

C, sleeve gastrectomy

I had a very supportive GP, who could see that my weight was not only having an impact on my physical well-being, but also my emotional.

K, gastric bypass

Most people, given the choice, would want to have their surgery through the NHS for reasons of cost together with good support and follow-up. In deciding who should, and who shouldn't, have weight loss surgery under the NHS, the primary care trusts (PCTs), who manage health funding, broadly follow guidelines laid down by the National Institute for Health and Clinical Excellence (NICE).[1] NICE looks at all the evidence for the effectiveness of medical treatments, including medication and surgery, and produces guidelines on when these treatments should be offered to patients. The initial 2002 NICE guidance on obesity surgery was replaced in 2006 by a broader guidance on the prevention and management of obesity in children and adults, which outlines the circumstances in which patients may be considered for surgery.

NICE suggests that weight loss surgery should be considered if:

- The patient has a BMI of 40 or more, or a BMI of 35–39 together with significant comorbidities. Comorbidities are health problems related to the obesity, such as type 2 diabetes, coronary heart disease, sleep apnoea, a history of stroke or transient ischaemic attacks (TIA) that are likely to be improved by weight loss. There is information about weight-related comorbidities in Chapter 3.
- All appropriate non-surgical measures (including diet and exercise) have failed to produce or maintain clinically beneficial weight loss for at least six months.
- The patient is receiving specialist, intensive weight management support.
- The patient is generally fit for surgery and anaesthesia.
- He or she is committed to the need for long-term follow-up.
- Finally, weight loss surgery may be considered as a first-line option for adults with a BMI of over 50, that is they may not have to demonstrate a history of diet attempts.

While some PCTs still follow these NICE guidelines when deciding funding, others have placed stricter criteria for who is eligible for weight loss surgery. Some areas only offer surgery to people with a BMI over 50 or a BMI of 45–50 with comorbidities that are sufficiently severe as to have a significant impact on their ability to carry out day-to-day activities. Some areas appear to only fund patients who have an extremely high BMI (60+). In addition, NHS services will expect you to have shown extensive efforts to lose weight through diet and exercise and pharmacological therapy (such as treatment with Orlistat), as well as a strong commitment to stick to the demands of surgery and attend regular follow-up appointments.

Research[2] shows that the lowest rates of complications are associated with surgery in bariatric centres that deal with high numbers of patients each year (over 100 patients compared with under 50 patients). In addition, high risk patients, such as older and very young patients, those with a BMI over 55, and patients with significant heart or respiratory problems, should have surgery at a high volume specialist centre, as should patients needing *revisional* surgery (that is, secondary bariatric surgery carried out when the initial surgery has failed to produce adequate weight loss or has caused ongoing problems).[3] Your NHS service should be willing to provide you with information about the number of patients they treat together with the surgeon's personal level of experience. There are no performance tables for bariatric surgeons in the UK, but you can learn more about surgeons and the hospitals where they work from the Dr Foster website, which was set up in collaboration with the Department of Health to provide the public with information about the availability and performance of local NHS and private healthcare services.

Going private?

In order to have weight loss surgery privately in the UK you will still need to meet NICE criteria, but you will not have to sit though the uncertainty of a prolonged NHS funding process and the surgeon will have shorter waiting times. Private weight loss surgery patients tend to have a lower BMI than NHS funded patients.[4]

If you are having surgery privately you will need to consider what surgeon to use, how much it will cost and the follow-up support offered. The prices for private weight loss surgery in the UK from the major providers are reasonably consistent, so a gastric bypass will cost £10,000–£12,000, a gastric band £6,000–£8,000 and a gastric balloon £4,000–£5,000. The gastric band is by far the most common bariatric procedure performed in the private sector. The sleeve gastrectomy is less available privately in the UK, but will cost around £10,000–£11,000, while biliopancreatic diversion/duodenal switch is not generally available.

The most important question to ask if you are contemplating going privately is not the price but what is included in the price, and you'll need to check what the package includes in terms of pre- and post-surgery care and support. Does the cost include thorough assessment with the surgeon, dietitian and physician or endocrinologist, including any scans and tests before surgery? The assessment is an important opportunity for you to consider whether surgery is the right decision and it is important that the process allows you time to reflect on your decision. For this reason you need to be wary of private services, in the UK or abroad, that seem to offer only a cursory assessment or that give you little opportunity to think about your decision. You need thinking space to be ready for surgery and a surgeon who suggests admission just days or weeks after a brief consultation is not allowing you time to make the necessary emotional and dietetic preparations.

> [I] telephoned the company and the assessment was organised for two weeks later. [The] deposit was taken on the initial telephone call . . . I saw the nurse practitioner, patient coordinator and the nurse who took my medical readings . . . I didn't know I wouldn't be seeing the consultant.
>
> A, gastric band

> [The private surgeon] agreed my surgery on first visit and informed me of the pros and cons, but was . . . not interested in side effects. He just assured me I would lose 5 st . . . [I got] OK [information about] pre op and post to six weeks, but no support long-term about effects on digestion, vitamin and mineral requirements, [whether] I would gain weight again, etc.
>
> J, sleeve gastrectomy

Services can vary considerably in the support and follow-up package that is included. Check what happens if your stay in hospital is extended by complications and whether you are covered for additional corrective surgery if anything goes wrong. If you are having a gastric band, how many band fills are included in the cost? Do they provide ongoing support after surgery, such as access to a specialist multidisciplinary team, a local support group or telephone helpline?

The package from a private clinic should include (as a minimum) any scans or tests needed prior to surgery, surgical cover in case of complications and access to specialist surgical and dietetic support. With the gastric band you should be able to access unlimited band fills for at least two years. You should be given a consultation with the surgeon and dietitian, and ideally should be asked if you want a meeting with a psychologist or counsellor to discuss any issues relating to your emotional health and eating habits that could affect the success of surgery.

> Considering I went private, the service I anticipated wasn't quite up to the mark. To be frank it was . . . in you go, let's see your money . . . and now you can go home.
>
> A, gastric band

It may be cheaper if you go to abroad for surgery; surgical services in Belgium and Turkey, for example, offer gastric bypass and bands for around half the price you'd pay in the UK, but you may receive limited post-surgical support and will have to pay upwards of £100 for each band fill. The value of the gastric band is in its flexibility and adjustability, so you are likely to need a fair number of fills before you hit the right level. You will also need to consider whether you can access dietetic or surgical help, and you may find yourself needing to pay a great deal extra if you have complications requiring a longer hospital stay or further surgery. You also will need to calculate additional costs of travelling for follow-up appointments. There may be an arrangement for you to see a surgeon in the UK for follow-ups and band fills, but these consultations are likely to be expensive. Many NHS and private services in the UK are reluctant to take on the follow-up care of patients who have had surgery abroad.

Weight loss surgery for young people

Extremely overweight children and adolescents are at risk of major health problems, such as type 2 diabetes, sleep apnoea and high blood pressure[5] and, as they go into adulthood, premature death.[6] As with adult bariatric patients these teenagers often experience depression and binge eating problems[7] and have a poor quality of life.

It is relatively unusual for teenagers to be offered bariatric surgery as it raises difficult issues about choice and consent and there is little information about potential long-term impact on emotional health, metabolic function and nutritional status.[8] Much less is known about the physical, psychological and social consequences of weight loss surgery for teenagers compared to adult patients, so it is essential that they have a careful assessment of need and, when surgery is offered, intensive, long-term support for themselves and their family. For this reason few doctors feel it is appropriate to refer children under the age of 15 years and one US survey found that nearly half of family doctors and paediatricians would never consider referring a child or teenager under the age of 18 for weight loss surgery.[9]

Surgery is restricted to those teenagers who have already developed comorbidities or where their emotional health or quality of life is severely affected by the weight and will only be considered if the young person is severely obese and all attempts at mainstream treatment, including at least six months of intensive dietary, exercise and behaviour change support, have been unsuccessful.

Recent recommendations[10] suggest that in order to consider surgery the young person should:

- be at least 15 years old
- have reached the final stages of puberty and is near or at their adult height
- have a BMI over 40, together with severe comorbidities such as type 2 diabetes, hypertension, non-fatty liver disease or obstructive sleep apnoea

- be able to understand the various treatment options and make an informed decision about surgery
- be motivated to make major lifestyle changes, are committed to ongoing support and follow-up and have the full support of their family.

Assessment should include investigation of any treatable causes of obesity and the physical, social and emotional factors that could affect the success of surgery. The bariatric team needs to have specialist paediatric expertise in psychological, social, medical, educational and family assessment. The young person and their family should be offered support and education about the potential risks of surgery and the necessary dietary and lifestyle changes and have access to ongoing follow-up support from the multidisciplinary team, including advice from dietitians, individualised nutritional supplementation and ongoing psychological help.[1]

The risks for adolescents, of surgical complications, poor weight loss and weight regain, are the same those faced by adults and less is known about the long-term impact on nutritional health, particularly with the gastric bypass. Some surgeons favour the gastric band for young people due to its lower risk profile and reversibility, but some teenagers are unable to tolerate it or show poor weight loss.[11]

Weight loss surgery is not considered suitable for teenagers who are unable to maintain the dietary changes and nutritional supplements; who are pregnant or breastfeeding; who have a drug or alcohol problem; who are seriously ill; or who have Prader-Willi syndrome, a congenital condition that causes the individual to overeat excessively (*hyperphagia*).[11] The teenager must be able to demonstrate that they understand the risks and be emotionally and intellectually mature enough to cope with the changes to their eating habits and lifestyle. Some experts question the capacity of teenagers, especially those under 13 years old, to make such a serious and life changing decision.[8] The support of the family, important for everyone undergoing weight loss surgery, is particularly so for teenagers and they will need to make a commitment to changes in their own diet and activity levels.

If you are an overweight teenager, or are worried about your son or daughter, the first step in getting support is talking to your GP who can advise you on treatment options.

What is my body mass index?

The NICE guidelines state that you need to have a BMI over 40 or a BMI of 35–39 together with other significant comorbidities before you can be considered for weight loss surgery.

Table 4.1 Body mass index (BMI) chart

Height	Normal weight BMI 23	Overweight BMI 29	Obese BMI 34	BMI 39	BMI 49	BMI 59	BMI 69
5′	55kg	68kg	79kg	91kg	114kg	137kg	160kg
5′3″	60kg	75kg	88kg	100kg	126kg	151kg	177kg
5′6″	65kg	82kg	96kg	110kg	138kg	166kg	194kg
5′9″	71kg	89kg	105kg	120kg	151kg	181kg	212kg
6′	77kg	98kg	114kg	133kg	164kg	197kg	231kg
6′3″	84kg	105kg	124kg	142kg	178kg	214kg	251kg

BMI is a measure of your weight in kilograms by your height in metres. Table 4.1 gives you a rough guide to your current BMI. First, find your height on the left hand side then look across to your nearest weight – this will give your BMI range. There are many BMI calculators online that will calculate your exact BMI, including a user-friendly version at www.nhs.uk/tools.

Do I meet the NICE criteria for weight loss surgery?

You should now have some idea as to whether you fit the criteria for weight loss surgery. Your next step is to make an appointment to speak

1. I have a BMI of 40 or more.   Yes ☐   No ☐
   or I have a BMI of 35–39.   Yes ☐   No ☐

   plus, I have been diagnosed with *at least one* of the following:

   Type 2 diabetes   ☐
   Sleep apnoea   ☐
   Coronary heart disease   ☐
   High blood pressure   ☐
   Stroke or TIA   ☐
   Arthritis   ☐

2. I have had support to lose weight through non-surgical means (such as medication and/or a weight management programme), but was unable to achieve or maintain significant weight loss.   Yes ☐   No ☐

3. I understand the need for detailed assessment by the bariatric team and am willing to commit to regular follow-up meetings with the bariatric team.   Yes ☐   No ☐

to your GP who can talk you through the process and options. It will help if you have all the relevant information to hand, so take a few minutes to answer the questions on the previous page.

If you have answered yes to all of these questions you may fit the NICE criteria for weight loss surgery and are potentially eligible for surgery under the NHS. However, depending on your health area, there are different criteria for NHS funding; you need to speak with your GP to get a clear idea about the options available to you.

Am I ready for surgery?

What I hope will become clear while reading this book is that weight loss surgery, while greatly beneficial for many patients, is not right for everyone. It requires a commitment to transforming eating behaviours and lifestyle that not everyone can manage. Now that you have some sense of whether surgery might be right for you *from a medical point of view*, spend a little time considering the emotional and social factors that could also affect the decision.

'I wish things were different' vs. 'I will change this'

If you decide to have weight loss surgery, and you want to ensure it's successful, you are committing yourself to a lifetime of restricted eating with a focus on a maintaining a sensible, balanced diet. Making changes to health behaviours is never easy; whether giving up smoking, starting an exercise routine or eating more healthily, it's rarely straightforward and even those with the most determination and willpower are going to have times when they're tempted to give up. Undergoing weight loss surgery is particularly challenging because it requires you to make a whole set of changes at the same time – as well as dramatically transforming how and what you eat, you also need to plan and prepare for all meals in advance, keep a food diary (and possibly a weight loss journal), give up smoking before surgery (to reduce the risks of surgery), reduce or give up alcohol and increase activity levels.

The *stages of change model*[12] helps us understand the way people make health changes. The model suggests that there are five key stages that people move through as they approach and establish a change in behaviour. These stages are flexible and people may move through them at different rates, sometimes falling back or making a leap forward.

The five stages of change are:

1. *Precontemplation stage*. People in this stage do not consider the behaviour to be a problem, they tend to downplay any disadvantages of the behaviour and dismiss likely benefits of change. In the case

of smoking, this would be reflected in statements such as: 'My grandfather smoked 60 a day and he lived to 98'; 'The damage is done now, there's no point changing a habit of a lifetime'; and 'When I've tried to give up before I just felt worse, I couldn't stop coughing'. Perhaps if you are a smoker or an ex-smoker you will recognise these justifications.

2. *Contemplation stage.* The individual begins to acknowledge the problems associated with the behaviour (be it smoking or eating too much) and is aware of the potential impact on their health. They no longer feel immune from the effects of the behaviour and may start to think about making a change.

3. *Preparation stage.* The person begins to plan for the change. Again using smoking as an example, they may go to their GP to get nicotine patches, set a date for giving up and tell friends and family that they want to make the change.

4. *Action stage.* This stage is where the individual makes the change (so stops smoking, goes to the gym and so on), but is vulnerable to relapsing. Support and encouragement from friends and family is important at this point.

5. *Maintenance stage.* This is about keeping up the new behaviour. The longer the behaviour change is sustained the less likely the person is to relapse, but it may take many months or even years for the new way of being to feel really confident. If you have been a smoker or have seen loved ones try to quit, you will know that the urge to smoke can re-emerge many years later, particularly at times of stress. It is this long-term change in behaviour that offers real health benefits and is generally based on shifts in the way the individual thinks about the behaviour together with the establishment of alternative strategies.

At each stage the person is assessing the potential pros and cons of change as well as questioning their personal confidence in making the change. The way people think and talk about the change gives clues to where they are in the process of change.

During the assessment for weight loss surgery, your *readiness for change* will be evaluated by the bariatric team. They will want to know how you are thinking about your diet and activity levels, and will be looking for evidence that you recognise the need to change and that you have thought about how these changes will be managed.

How ready am I for change?

Look at the statements below and think about whether they apply to you. Do you agree with them strongly, only a little or not at all? Your answers should give you some idea of how psychologically ready you are to make healthy changes. Of course none of these questions can predict whether you can cope with the changes demanded by weight loss surgery, but they may help you consider whether you are able to take on the challenge:

1. The health risks associated with obesity are exaggerated.
2. By being overweight I am standing up against social norms about what's attractive.
3. I do not like other people telling me what I should eat.
4. My weight has benefits for me, e.g. in my relationships.
5. With surgery I won't have to make much effort to change my eating habits.
6. I worry about the effect on my family if I became ill.
7. I'm aware each day how much my weight affects my health and quality of life.
8. I know I need to make major changes to lose weight and sometimes feel overwhelmed by the thought of it.
9. At the moment I am unsure about how the benefits of surgery balance against the downsides.
10. I feel ready to make changes to my eating habits.
11. I want to eat to live not live to eat.
12. The weight is having such a negative impact on my health and quality of life; I know I can't go on as I have been.
13. I have made an effort to find out about the risks and benefits of weight loss surgery.
14. I have sought out people who have had surgery so I can hear about their experiences.
15. I have spoken to my family and friends about the need to change my eating habits.
16. At this time, I feel ready to make major changes to my diet and eating habits.
17. I have asked the family to get rid of all snack foods in the house.
18. I have started walking to work every day rather than using the car.

Statements 1–5: If you agree strongly with a number of these statements it suggests that you are in the precontemplation stage, that you do not believe your weight is a major problem for your well-being or do not feel there's much you can do about it. You may be seeing weight loss surgery as a magic cure rather than a *tool* to help you make changes to your eating. Maybe your decision to have surgery has been quite impulsive. You need to question whether surgery is right for you at this time; you may want to spend some time talking to other people, doing research on the internet or continuing to read through this book before you proceed further.

Statements 6–9: If you agree with these statements you may be in the contemplation stage. You know that your weight problem is negatively affecting your life, but may also feel unsure or overwhelmed by the thought of coping with the changes needed.

Statements 10–16: Agreement with these statements suggests you are in the preparation stage; you feel ready to make real changes and have started to lay the groundwork.

Statements 17–18: If you agree with these, it suggests that you are already in the action stage. You have made changes to your eating and exercise habits and feel committed to making the changes needed to improve your health.

My guess is that, as you have already read to the end of Chapter 4 in this book, many of you will be in the contemplation, preparation or action stages. You may feel extremely distressed about your weight and are looking to weight loss surgery as a solution to this. You may be at a point where you want change, but are frightened by the enormity of the decision or you may feel completely ready to take on the challenge.

Whatever the case for you, it's essential that you are aware that weight loss surgery is about *you* making changes. While everyone accepts that no one else can quit smoking, give up alcohol or go to the gym for them, they do not always see weight loss surgery in the same way. Some people believe that the success of weight loss surgery is down to the surgeon. While you definitely want a skilful surgeon, his or her job is insignificant compared to the years of work you must put in to make the process successful. Remember, the surgeon is operating on your stomach, he is not doing brain surgery and you will be left with the same personality, habits, strengths, weaknesses and difficulties you ever had.

Is the timing right?

Your readiness for change and your capacity to cope with the demands of surgery depend not just on your own determination and motivation, but also on what else is happening in your life. If you are facing major upheavals or stresses it will impact on the emotional and practical resources you have available to cope with surgery. Ideally you would undergo weight loss surgery when all other areas of your life – your family life, work and so on – are reasonably stable so you can focus your energies on coping with recovery from surgery and making the necessary changes to your diet and activity. Of course it's not always possible to ensure a stress-free space, but if you are experiencing a very turbulent or difficult time in your life it may be appropriate to delay surgery to give yourself the best chance of success.

Are you currently facing major life stresses? Have you experienced any of the following life challenges in the past year?

- Death of a loved one.
- A major change to your living circumstances.
- Health problems in yourself or your family.
- Ongoing stress at work or loss of work.
- Difficulties in your relationships with your spouse or partner, including separation or divorce.
- Worries about your children, e.g. health, schooling, behaviour.
- Legal problems.
- Significant money worries.

If you have been through one or more of these stresses in the past year or so, you will need to consider if it is the right time to go through surgery. These events can *use up* your coping capacity and leave you vulnerable to feeling overwhelmed. Whether or not you should delay surgery will depend on the number and severity of the stresses you have faced; the extent to which the stressful situations have been resolved; how much practical and emotional support you have from friends and family; and how well you have coped with stress in the past. Again this is about you making a realistic assessment of your ability to take on another major stress (i.e. surgery) and cope with an extended disruption to your normal life and routine. Most bariatric services are happy to delay surgery for a time and it is important to give yourself the best chance of making it a success.

What about the practicalities?

As well as having the right mental attitude, success with weight loss surgery also depends upon some basic practical requirements. The way you manage your mealtimes, the availability of meal breaks during your working day and access to cooking facilities are all important. Again, spend a few minutes thinking about the following questions:

- Do I find it easy to access the foods I need? Are there any social, physical or financial blocks to getting appropriate, nutritious food? Are there other people I can call on to help with shopping?
- Do I have adequate facilities at home for storing and preparing food (e.g. cooker, fridge/freezer, microwave, blender, etc.)?
- Does my home or work environment affect my ability to eat healthily (e.g. access to a work canteen that sells healthy food)?
- Do my employers allow me enough break time for a meal to be eaten slowly and carefully? (No more eating a sandwich at your desk while on the phone to clients!)

- Does my daily routine allow me time to engage in physical activity?
- Are there social, physical or financial blocks to regular physical activity (e.g. accommodation limits access to opportunities for exercise; the needs of other people at home; local access to parks, gym and swimming pool; the cost of swimming or joining the gym)? Have you thought about how you can overcome these blocks?
- Do I have people around who can offer practical support while I'm recovering after surgery?
- Do I have people around who will provide emotional support and encouragement in the months after surgery?

Throughout this section about psychological and practical readiness I have asked you to reflect on questions that could affect the outcome of weight loss surgery. These questions are likely to come up during the assessment for surgery, as discussed in the next chapter, and spending some time thinking through these issues will put you in a good position to make the right decision given your personal situation at this time. As explained by one gastric bypass patient, weight loss surgery is not for everyone:

> Do not just do it because you have seen it on television and think it looks good. You have to be really large, you have to have actually tried all the diets and solutions, you have to be committed to exercise and recognise your food choices may never be the same. As everyone will say too, IT IS ONLY A TOOL. It is not easy, it is not a quick fix, and even those who are very successful are often so at the price of bad bowels, regularly throwing up or a very limited diet. And you can cheat anything if you really want to.
>
> A, gastric bypass

5

Assessment for weight loss surgery

In this chapter we will consider what happens when you have been referred to a bariatric surgeon and are starting the assessment process. While the National Institute for Health and Clinical Excellence (NICE) guidelines are the *bottom line* – that is you cannot access surgery if you don't fulfil these criteria – they are only part of the picture. Ultimately the clinical assessment is less concerned with whether weight loss surgery is right for you (your GP has already made this judgement based on your weight and health problems) and is more concerned about whether you're right for weight loss surgery. So the purpose of the bariatric assessment is to determine whether you are a suitable candidate for surgery and whether you have a good chance of managing the change in lifestyle, achieving significant weight loss and benefiting from substantial improvements in your health and quality of life.

NICE guidelines[1] state that you are expected to undergo a comprehensive assessment of any psychological and medical factors that could affect the success of surgery, and that you understand the risks and benefits associated with surgery. NICE also emphasises that you should have a say in the choice of surgical intervention, through discussion with your surgeon and bariatric team, taking into account your medical, social and emotional needs.

The bariatric team will assess: your medical and surgical fitness for surgery; your eating habits and ability to stick to a healthy post-surgery diet; access to support from other people; and your emotional health. It may be the first time you've been encouraged to think about your weight journey – the factors that have influenced your weight gain and the nature of your eating habits. Some people, having been through the assessment, will choose not to have surgery or want to have another go at losing weight through diet and exercise before making a final decision. The assessment will offer better understanding of the risks and benefits of surgery and the impact on your day-to-day life, so by the end you should be in a good position to make an informed decision about this life-changing event.

> On reflection I can see it's important that people do not have surgery if they don't have the ability to use that tool effectively.
>
> N, gastric bypass

Surgical consultation

> [. . .] it was meeting with [the surgeon] that gave me the opportunity to have a proper dialogue and discussion on why/how/ what and if it would really work.
>
> A, gastric bypass

Bariatric surgeons understand the importance of selecting patients who will benefit most from weight loss surgery. The criteria for accessing weight loss surgery have been set by NICE, the UK government health advisory body, which require that: you should have a body mass index (BMI) of 40 or over, or a BMI between 35 and 39.9 and suffer from a obesity-related health problems, such as type 2 diabetes, hypertension, sleep apnoea or dyslipidaemia; you should have tried other weight loss treatments without permanent success; you should have a reasonable understanding of the procedure; you are well motivated to make the lifestyle changes required to be successful; and that you are fit for anaesthesia.

The surgeon will talk you through your medical history including previous surgery and will examine you to ensure that your body is suitable for surgery. He/she will want to know about your general health, history of weight gain, eating habits and alcohol use and will make a broad assessment of your emotional capacity to cope with surgery, as well as your understanding and expectations of surgery. It's important to remember that when your consultant talks about your ideal weight or healthy weight they are talking about weight loss that would produce health benefits, not necessarily what you'd like to weigh. Your ideal weight – the weight that you think would make you feel confident, fit and happy – is not necessarily what's offered by weight loss surgery.

On the basis of the assessment the surgeon will decide whether you also need to be seen by an anaesthetist, endocrinologist or psychologist for further review.

> He asked what I understood about weight loss surgery and what type of operation I thought I wanted . . . I needed to write a letter of commitment to confirm that I wanted to go ahead with the

process . . . we discussed how I was getting on with what the dietitian had put in place, I was examined fully and they explained that due to my high BMI I may end up with a gastric sleeve rather than a bypass.

C, sleeve gastrectomy

[The surgeon] . . . told me I had been accepted for surgery [and] explained what this meant, what would happen, and what I could expect afterwards. He clearly explained the pros and cons and the risks involved in the operation. I felt I understood exactly what to expect and what they would expect of me.

K, gastric bypass

The decision as to the best bariatric procedure should be based on discussion between yourself and the surgeon. He/she may well have a view on the most appropriate surgical procedure, but you also need to be sure that you understand the procedure and are willing to accept the potential risks. However much you feel at the end of your tether it is important to think carefully about the choices available to you and remember that it is you, and not the surgeon, who will have to live with the surgery.

The surgeon recommended the sleeve . . . I was so desperate I went along with it, I felt so ill and depressed I was willing to take the risk based on 'could I feel any worse?' and if I died maybe it would be a blessing.

J, sleeve gastrectomy

Dietetic assessment

The most helpful thing was not being judged because I ate the wrong food.

C, sleeve gastrectomy

The dietitian will consider whether you are able to reflect on your weight gain over the years and understand the factors and events that have influenced your eating behaviour. You will be questioned about your past attempts to manage your weight and may be asked to write a list of all your diet attempts and how successful they were; this gives the team an idea about your ability to maintain a restricted diet over a period of time. The dietitian will ask in detail about your eating habits and triggers for overeating. Different aspects of eating behaviour such as food preferences, portion sizes, snacking and the structure of mealtimes will be considered. He/she will assess where excess calories are coming from and ask about episodes of disordered or uncontrolled eating.

> [Before surgery] I would snack a lot. I would turn to food for almost any reason; happy sad, in pain, stress – [food] was my comfort, my best friend.
>
> J, gastric bypass

The dietitian may suggest you start a food diary to develop a better understanding of the factors that affect your eating. Recording everything you eat and drink each day increases your awareness of eating habits, enhances control, supports you in making changes to your diet, and allows you to monitor positive changes. You may decide to start a food diary before you see the dietitian and there is one you can use as a guide at the end of this chapter.

> The dietitian goes through your food questionnaire with you . . . asks you all sorts of questions regarding your lifestyle, past and present . . . about your eating habits, and reasons you think that you have reached this point . . . [They] also give you a food diary for one week. I was dishonest in mine. I didn't write down everything I had eaten, I was embarrassed, and I admitted this to the dietitian. She was understanding, but explained that without all the information, the team don't know the full picture.
>
> K, gastric bypass

The dietitian will also consider practical issues that could impact on outcome, such as access to cooking facilities, cooking skills and time constraints. They will talk you through the pre-surgery diet and provide detailed information about the diet you will need to follow after surgery, including the food and drink you'll need to avoid. You may be asked about your hopes and expectations of surgery and access to social support. You may be encouraged to attend a patient support group to talk to other patients to gain a better understanding of the reality of living with weight loss surgery.

Medical/endocrinology assessment

In many bariatric services, patients will be seen by an endocrinologist or physician and you are more likely to require this assessment if you have diabetes. An endocrinologist is a doctor specialised in disorders of the hormone systems, such as diabetes, thyroid disease, metabolic disorders, menopause, polycystic ovaries and so on.

The endocrinologist or physician will be looking for medical causes of obesity, such as Cushing's syndrome (when weight gain results from excess levels of cortisol that can result from a number of different medical conditions), requiring treatment in its own right. For this they may carry out an overnight *dexamethasone suppression test;* you are given a dose of dexamethasone to take around 11 p.m. and blood is taken first thing in the morning to measure cortisol levels. This test allows the doctor to identify Cushing's syndrome and helps to diagnose the likely cause.

The endocrinologist or physician will also be looking at the medication you are taking. If they feel any medication is contributing to your weight gain they may ask the prescribing doctor to look into this. If you're diabetic they will look at your medical regimen and consider how well your blood sugars are controlled. When you have surgery (or when you start the pre-surgery diet) your diabetes medication may need to be modified and the endocrinologist will advise your GP or diabetic team accordingly.

You will be asked about symptoms of heartburn, reflux and indigestion which may indicate the presence of a hiatus hernia. If you have these symptoms you may have a barium swallow or gastroscopy (where a camera is inserted into the stomach). A hiatus hernia occurs when a part of the stomach has moved through an opening in the diaphragm (the sheet of muscle that divides the abdominal space from the chest space) causing heartburn. This kind of hernia can sometimes be fixed at the same time as the bariatric procedure.

You may be given a questionnaire asking about your daytime sleepiness levels to screen for obstructive sleep apnoea. If the endocrinologist thinks you may have sleep apnoea he/she will recommend referral for further investigations at the respiratory clinic. You may also require a breathing capacity test and heart trace or scan to assess your general anaesthetic risk.

In addition to these medical factors, the endocrinologist will be considering whether you have realistic expectations of surgery and understand the amount of effort and change needed to make surgery successful. As with all members of the team they will be thinking about which bariatric procedure is best for you given your weight, medical needs and eating habits.

Psychology assessment

Many surgeons want their patients to see a psychologist or psychiatrist before surgery to assess your capacity to cope with the changes to diet and lifestyle required by weight loss surgery and your commitment to long-term follow up; to check that you understand fully the risks and benefits of surgery; and to identify any mental health problems or eating habits that could impact on your success with surgery. The purpose of the psychology review is to ensure, as far as possible, that the procedure is likely to be safe and effective for you. The psychology assessment will consider in detail your eating habits, your mood and any history of psychological difficulties or trauma, as well as wanting to know about your strategies for coping with stress and the social support you can access from family and friends. The aim is not to exclude people from surgery, but to ensure that you have access to appropriate help and support.

> Meeting the psychologist . . . I was so nervous. I was also quite tearful. She was so kind and understanding, and completely put me at my ease, she told me that everything that was discussed was not a trick question, there are no wrong and right answers, each person is different.
>
> K, gastric bypass

Emotional health

A significant number of people who seek weight loss surgery have had emotional difficulties at some point in their life, mainly problems with depression or anxiety.[2] Somewhere between 50–85 per cent of people seeking weight loss surgery will have had a diagnosis of depression at some point in their life,[3] 40 per cent have a current mental health problem, most commonly depression and anxiety[4] and a third have more than one psychiatric diagnosis.[5] As many as a quarter of weight loss surgery patients have a diagnosis of personality disorder.[6] Personality disorders are long-standing and pronounced problems in behaviour and thinking that affect the individual's emotional experience, the way they think about the world, and their relationships with other people. People with personality disorders often have problems with impulse control so are at risk of self-harming behaviours and may struggle to take adequate care of their health and dietary needs after surgery.

As we saw in Chapter 3 there are a number of reasons why obesity can lead to depression, as the result of social stigma, isolation, body dissatisfaction, lowered self-esteem and diminished quality of life, but some people experience depression or other emotional difficulties before the onset of obesity, which may have contributed to weight gain. In these cases weight loss surgery alone is unlikely to resolve the emotional health problems. So while weight loss surgery generally helps people to feel better[7] it is not a treatment for mental health problems and psychiatric treatment should not be delayed in the expectation of a spontaneous improvement after surgery.[8]

The psychology assessment is guided by an understanding of the issues that have been linked with a less successful outcome. While you may view surgery as a *last chance,* those who fail to lose a good amount of weight, who are unable to tolerate the side effects or are otherwise dissatisfied with their surgery outcome, appear to be at particular risk of a deterioration in mood and there is evidence of increased risk of suicide after weight loss surgery.[9]

Tom Stevens and his colleagues[10] have developed a traffic light system as a framework for assessing the risk of people encountering problems after surgery. Red indicates that the patient is not suitable for weight loss surgery, amber indicates that they may be suitable but are at higher risk and may need additional support before or after surgery, while green indicates that the patient is a good candidate for surgery.

Red light

People who have ongoing, poorly controlled psychotic illness, such schizophrenia or bipolar disorder; current drug or alcohol dependency; a history of serious self-neglect or self-harm; or significant learning disabilities or dementia, are not considered suitable for surgery as they are unlikely to be able to tolerate and comply with the post-surgical restrictions. People with a history of serious mental health problems or personality disorder may be required to have ongoing support from a psychiatrist or their local community mental health team and would be expected to have had no psychiatric admissions or episodes of self-harm in the previous year. Being depressed or anxious in itself does not seem to be associated with a poorer outcome with weight loss surgery, but there is some indication that having more than one psychiatric disorder is linked to less than ideal weight loss.[4]

Patients with a history of drug or alcohol problems are generally expected to have been abstinent for at least one year. As the mal-absorptive procedures, gastric bypass and biliopancreatic diversion/duodenal switch, affect the way alcohol is processed by the body[11] they are not recommended for people who have a history of alcohol abuse.[10]

Amber light

An amber light indicates that a person could be at risk of emotional or medical difficulties after surgery and so may need additional support. This would include people who have struggled with mental health problems in the past, but who are now stable; a past history of drug or alcohol use; a history of eating disorders; mild learning disabilities; an ongoing binge eating disorder (see below for more information about disordered eating); and people who have struggled to follow medical advice in the past or who show poor motivation for change.

Green light

The psychologist will be looking for evidence of motivation, realistic expectations and ability to manage the post-surgery diet. Good candidates for surgery will show high levels of motivation and be realistic in their expectations of surgery. They will have an understanding of the causes of their weight gain and will have reasonably stable eating habits.

It may be tempting to conceal some emotional or mental health issues from the bariatric psychologist, especially if it feels that weight loss surgery is your last chance. This is not helpful in the long run as it stops you accessing the help you need to make surgery successful. These guidelines have been developed because these factors have been linked to problems in coping with the demands of surgery and increase the possibility of complications that could have a negative effect on

Table 5.1 The traffic light system for assessing psychological risk factors[10]

RED *not currently suitable for surgery*	AMBER *may need additional help and support*	GREEN *suitable for surgery*
Severe unstable mental health problems such as schizophrenia and bipolar disorder.	History of severe mental illness that has been stable for at least 12 months with no psychiatric hospital admissions or episodes of self-harm within this time.	No history of severe mental health problems.
Ongoing alcohol or drug dependency problem.	History of drug or alcohol dependency.	No history of drug or alcohol dependency.
Active bulimia nervosa.	History of eating disorder or current binge eating disorder. Poor understanding of eating behaviours.	Regular balanced diet. Good understanding of eating habits and causes of weight gain.
Severe or moderate learning disability or a diagnosis of dementia or other significant cognitive impairment.	Mild learning disability.	Good understanding of the procedure and potential risks.
Current non-compliance with treatment (e.g. not taking medication according to the doctor's instructions).	Non-attendance or poor compliance with previous treatments. Poor motivation. Unrealistic expectations of surgery.	Good motivation and realistic expectations of surgery. Good compliance with treatment.
Severe personality disorder.	History of personality disorder where the patient is able to demonstrate sustained changes to problematic behaviours including self-harm.	

your health and quality of life. In all cases the psychological risk factors will be considered alongside the likely medical benefits and where possible the team should help you access the further support or treatment you need.

If you have difficulties that could impact on the success of surgery, the bariatric team may recommend referral on to other services for further help and support prior to surgery. This could include your local mental health team, community weight management service, eating disorders team, drug and alcohol service, psychological therapy or counselling service, 'exercise on prescription' scheme, or a pain management programme if your chronic pain problem is having a significant effect on your ability to exercise.

Remember, you want weight loss surgery because you hope it will be successful – that you will lose a substantial amount of weight and have a longer, healthier and happier life. This is also what your bariatric team wants; they will recommend you for surgery if they think you have a reasonable chance of achieving success.

Binge eating disorder and other disordered eating

Binge eating disorder

A relatively high number of patients seeking weight loss surgery have a problem with binge eating[12,13] often dating back to childhood.[14] A binge episode is characterised by the consumption of an excessive amount of food in a relatively short period of time with the individual experiencing a loss of control over their eating. During a binge you feel unable to stop eating; you may eat rapidly, barely tasting the food. Some people pace the floor while having a binge episode and hide the evidence of the binge from others. While it's happening the experience of eating can be pleasurable or you may feel numb, but this feeling is quickly replaced by a sense of shame or disgust.

If binge episodes happen frequently (at least twice a week) and cause distress, the person is said to have a *binge eating disorder*.[15] People seeking weight loss surgery are more likely to meet the criteria for binge eating disorder than, for example, a similar group of people attending a community slimming club.[16] Binge eating disorder is associated with higher rates of emotional difficulties such as depression, anxiety, lower levels of happiness, poor self-esteem[2] and body image distress. It is thought that between 20 and 30 per cent of weight loss surgery candidates have a severe binge eating disorder, with up to two-thirds showing occasional binge eating.[14,17,18]

I ignored my diabetes and ate what I wanted. I was able to kid myself that I didn't overeat, but I did. I binged on certain foods.

I felt guilty every time I put food in my mouth. I was ashamed of my hunger and my need for the comfort of eating.

K, gastric bypass

I would shop on a Tuesday and have a 'food party' with all the food I had bought, almost to the point of being sick, but not quite, and still have a full evening meal when my husband got home.

J, sleeve gastrectomy

If you regularly try to get rid of calories consumed during a binge episode, for example by vomiting, laxatives or excessive exercise (known as compensatory behaviours), the diagnosis would be *bulimia* (or *bulimia nervosa*). Some weight loss surgery patients have a history of bulimia and the bariatric team would expect this to have been absent for at least 12 months before proceeding with surgery.

The central issue with binge episodes, and the factor that seems to have the most negative impact on individuals, is not the amount of food eaten or the frequency of binges, but the experience of loss of control[16] and it is this loss of control that people often want to contain through surgery. However, the experience of loss of control of eating can continue after surgery and has been associated with poorer weight loss and greater risk of weight regain.[19]

As an overall group, most studies suggest that people diagnosed with binge eating disorder do not show any difference in weight loss than non-binge eaters. However, they are more at risk of post-surgical loss of control and *grazing;* in the 12 months following surgery, as many as two-thirds of bariatric patients with a pre-surgery binge eating disorder report ongoing issue with grazing, and almost 50 per cent still have episodes of loss of control of eating[16] and these patients are more vulnerable to significant weight regain in the years following surgery.[20]

Night eating syndrome (NES)

Another form of disordered eating occurs when people eat significant amounts of food during the evening or night. NES is usually defined as a person eating more than a quarter of their overall calorie intake after the evening meal and/or wake during the night to eat at least twice a week. The individual is aware of and distressed by the behaviour[21] and, like binge eating disorder, NES is associated with depression.[22] NES is five times more common among very overweight people compared with the normal weight population[23] and it has been estimated that 20–30 per cent of bariatric patients, more often men, have symptoms of night eating before surgery.[16,24]

While there is no definitive research on the impact of NES on weight loss surgery outcome, at least one study suggests that pre-surgery night eating does not significantly affect weight loss or eating behaviour after surgery,[16] but as with binge eating it is likely to result in less than optimum weight loss if continued after surgery.

> I'd wake up around 3 a.m. and creep downstairs so as not to wake up my family. I'd want to have just a little snack to get rid of the hunger so I could get back to sleep, but once I started eating I found it hard to stop. I'd eat chocolate, toast, crisps, ham . . . anything else that was around. I would go shopping the next day to stock up the cupboard so my husband wouldn't know.

Emotional eating and grazing

> I had the best will power in the world until problems occurred at home and I was stressed. Then . . . I just grabbed things as and when I could.
>
> A, gastric band

Less intense than binge eating, but still making you vulnerable to gaining weight, emotional eating is a tendency to use food as a way of suppressing or coping with difficult emotions. Around 40 per cent of bariatric patients identify emotional eating as a cause of pre-surgical weight gain.[25] Grazing is characterised by periods of near continuous eating which may or may not be emotionally driven. Grazing may involve consuming very large amounts of food, like a binge episode, but takes place over a longer period of time. It is associated with less dietary restraint, greater disinhibition of eating and higher levels of subjective hunger. It has been suggested that a quarter of weight loss surgery patients show a pattern of grazing before surgery and there is a significant risk of this continuing after surgery. Grazing post-surgery is linked to poorer weight loss and more depression.[16]

Are you an emotional eater? The Boston Interview for Bariatric Surgery by Sogg and Mori (2008)[26] asks:

- Do you frequently eat in response to negative emotions?
- Do you find that you frequently use food as a coping mechanism?
- Do you find that you frequently use food to calm or 'medicate' yourself?
- Are your current emotions or stressors contributing to your weight by causing you to eat more?
- Do you feel that eating in response to emotions contributes significantly to your weight or makes it difficult to lose weight?

I comfort ate when I was bored or when I was upset or stressed . . .
I often rewarded myself with sweets and thought nothing of eating
a 200g bar of chocolate in front of the telly.

N, gastric bypass

If you are someone who regularly uses food as a way of managing
stress or upset, you will need to think about how you will manage this
after surgery. If it is your primary coping strategy, surgery would
remove an important prop, you will be unable to use food in this way
and so it may leave you feeling vulnerable. There are suggestions in
Chapter 6 on how you can develop new emotional coping skills.

Impact of disordered eating on outcome

We do not yet fully understand the impact of disordered eating on the
outcome of weight loss surgery and research finding have been incon-
clusive.[15] Some studies have indicated that binge eating resolves after
surgery and has no significant impact on the success of surgery. Other
studies have found the people with a binge disorder lose less weight
after surgery than patients without a binge eating disorder. Generally
the more long-term the study, the more likely they are to find a difference in weight loss between bingers and non-bingers.[20] While we may
not be very good at predicting exactly who will do well with surgery, it
seems pretty clear that people's reaction to the changed relationship
with food after surgery determines how well they do.

In the months after surgery the small stomach pouch effectively
prevents you from consuming large amounts of food, but problematic
eating can reoccur later. One to two years after surgery it is normal for
the constraints of surgery to ease off; you may start to experience less
food restriction, increased hunger and a greater tolerance for a range
of foods. It is at this stage that you are most vulnerable to falling back
into old patterns of relating to food. Your response to food and ability to
maintain a stable and healthy eating pattern at this point will determine the ultimate outcome of surgery and a re-emergence of emotional
eating, grazing or binging can lead to weight regain.

So, if you have disordered eating before surgery it does not necessarily mean that you will show less weight loss, but if uncontrolled
eating occurs after surgery, even if you are not eating the large amounts
you were before, this can mean less than ideal weight loss in the longer
term,[19] and disordered eating has been associated with complications
following gastric band, including band slippage, erosion and dilation of
the stomach pouch.[27]

If you are having regular binge episodes or are an emotional
eater you should speak to your bariatric team. While it is not seen as
a definite 'red light' it could affect how well you manage with the

post-surgery diet and how much weight you lose. Depending on the frequency or severity of the binge episodes or other problematic eating, your bariatric team may suggest that you receive some psychological support to manage this behaviour before going ahead with surgery. However, some experts believe that, even if long-term weight loss is not as good as it should be, surgery is still likely for most people to give a better outcome than no surgery[28] and that psychological treatment for binge eating should occur *after* surgery if it becomes a problem.

Social support

> I have a fantastic support network from my husband and family, which cannot be underestimated as this would be a very hard thing to do alone.
>
> K, gastric bypass

As weight loss surgery is a stressful event requiring major changes to your lifestyle, it is important that you have good support from family and friends, who can provide practical help immediately after surgery as well as ongoing encouragement. People with good support from others tend to do better, losing more weight than those with less robust support[29] and reporting better quality of life.[30]

Of course, not everyone thinking about weight loss surgery receives a positive response from the people around them. Some believe, incorrectly, that weight loss surgery is somehow 'cheating' – that people should just apply more willpower and lose the excess weight by dieting. Family members may feel threatened by the thought of their loved one losing weight, fearing that it will change them or alter the relationship. Friends or family who are also overweight may feel envious. Many people are naturally concerned about the surgical risk for their loved one and will be reassured by information about the real risks and benefits of surgery, but others are not be so easily appeased and may continue to express negative attitudes. Talking openly to your partner about the impact of the weight loss is vital. Your partner may need reassurance that losing weight won't lead you to seek a new relationship and in general the research indicates that marital relationships improve after surgery.[31]

Problems at home, marital conflict, divorce, difficulties with children, caring for elderly or disabled relatives, a recent move of house, can all impact on the support you have available from others. During assessment the team will enquire about access to support and may ask whether you anticipate anyone reacting badly to your weight loss. If you are concerned about this issue you should discuss it with the team before surgery. Remember also that many people find the support available from patient support groups or online forums of great help, and there's information about where to find these in Chapter 11.

What happens if I am not in a positive, supportive relationship?

Support from those close to you is essential during the adjustment to life after weight loss surgery and you may want to reflect on the impact of your relationship on your capacity to cope with these demands. Unfortunately some partners are not able to offer adequate support because of their own health or emotional problems. The psychology assessment may be a helpful opportunity to think about the effect of your personal situation on your ability to handle surgery. Do you have sufficient physical and emotional resources left over from caring for your partner (and others . . . children, parents?) to look after yourself after surgery? If you are primary carer for your partner you will need to talk together about who will take over their care, as well as who is available to support you, in the initial weeks.

Some people are unwilling to offer support with major life changes or feel threatened by the prospect of their partner losing weight and becoming more attractive to others. This refusal to help may be deliberate and malicious or unconscious, driven by anxiety, but either way potentially threatens your chances of success. If your partner has been highly insecure or controlling within the relationship or has previously sabotaged your diet attempts, this raises more concerns and could be a threat to the success of surgery.

If you feel this could be the case in your relationship, ask yourself:

- Has my partner failed to support my efforts/goals whole-heartedly in the past?
- Has my partner sabotaged my attempts to diet by bringing home snacks or encouraging me to eat foods I shouldn't?
- Does my partner often feel insecure about our relationship? Does he/she accuse me of having affairs unfairly?
- Has my partner's insecurity become more pronounced when I've lost weight in the past?
- Does my partner stop me going out to see friends or family?
- Does my partner control what I wear and where I go?
- Is my partner physically or emotionally abusive?
- Does my partner have a drug or alcohol problem?

If you answered yes to one or more of these questions, you will need to consider whether it is possible for you to cope successfully with the challenges of weight loss surgery in the context of your relationship. This relationship, if it remains unchanged, is unlikely to offer the conditions necessary for positive change in your life. If possible you need to seek support from your family and friends and in some circumstances it may be appropriate for you and your partner to have relationship counselling.

If you are isolated from others or in a problematic or abusive relationship talk to your GP and bariatric team about getting support. Information about other sources of support and advice can be found in Chapter 11.

Compliance with treatment

Weight loss surgery requires you to follow specific dietary guidelines, take vitamins and minerals daily and attend follow-up appointments with the bariatric team. A failure to stick to the *rules* after surgery can lead to serious medical complications.

For this reason the clinical team will be concerned with your capacity to comply with medical treatment and follow medical advice consistently. A history of repeated non-attendance at hospital appointments or evidence of poor compliance with a medical regime (for example, not taking your insulin as advised or failing to use continuous positive airway pressure (CPAP) regularly) may be seen as a potential contraindication for surgery.

Expectations of surgery

Throughout the assessment, the bariatric team will consider whether you have a good understanding of the bariatric procedure, that you fully understand the risks and benefits, and are realistic in what you expect from surgery. In one American study, almost 100 per cent of assessing psychologists/psychiatrists considered poor understanding or unrealistic expectations to be a *definite* or *possible* contraindication for surgery.[32]

Many, many patients say they will take the weight loss offered by surgery and then, *through additional personal effort with diet and exercise*, will lose more weight. In reality this *extra effort* you'll use to push for further weight loss is, in fact, the effort you need to make to get the weight loss your bariatric surgeon is talking about. You need to understand and acknowledge that, after relatively rapid weight loss in the first 18 months or so after surgery, weight loss slows down and you may have some weight regain. Weight loss surgery does not get you down to a normal weight and you may still be significantly overweight. Your ability to eat and drink normally has been permanently removed, and you are likely to have a problem with excess skin. Losing weight may not give you everything you wish for. While it will hopefully improve your health and mobility, it will not resolve all of life's problems – it will not stop you becoming depressed or having difficult relationships or make you socially confident if you weren't before, and it will certainly not improve your finances or make your children behave better. Human beings are very vulnerable to *if only* thinking and many patients have unrealistic hopes and dreams about how surgery will change their lives. If you don't reflect on these hopes, and keep them in check, you are in danger of being disappointed and demoralised a couple of years down the line and we know that this can be associated with depression, problematic eating habits and weight regain.

In one study[33] of people's hopes of surgery, the majority of patients greatly overestimated their probable weight loss. Despite having attended an educational group, patients stated that they would be *happy* with a weight loss of 85 per cent excess weight and would find *acceptable* a weight loss of 74 per cent excess weight. As bariatric surgery offers an average weight loss of around 60 per cent excess weight[34] this leaves scope for a lot of very unhappy folk. Interestingly, in the same study, people *underestimated* the beneficial impact of surgery on their health. This mismatch between expectations and outcome suggests that weight loss surgery should perhaps be rebranded as *metabolic surgery* – for the treatment of diabetes, coronary heart disease, sleep apnoea and so on – with weight loss simply being a *side effect* of the procedure.

How much weight will I lose?

As we can see unrealistic expectations of weight loss can cause distress and frustration after surgery, so it is helpful to work out roughly what degree of weight loss to expect. It has been shown that across all procedures patients lose *on average* 60 per cent of their excess weight (that is, 60 per cent of the difference between your current weight and your ideal weight – often written as 60 per cent EWL) though this depends on the procedure you have (the gastric band offers around 50 per cent excess weight loss (EWL)) and not all patients lose this amount of weight.

You maximum weight loss is generally seen a year or two post-surgery and then there is the possibility of some weight regain. Six years after surgery more than three-quarters of gastric bypass patients maintain a weight loss of 50 per cent excess weight or more[35] which means that upwards of 20 per cent of patients have been left with excess weight loss of *less* than 50 per cent. By ten years after surgery, average weight loss maintained is 25 per cent total pre-surgery weight for gastric bypass and 14 per cent for gastric band.[36] While this is much better weight loss than most people could realistically expect without surgery (over ten years, a matched group of people who that didn't have surgery show an average weight gain), nevertheless it may not be the dramatic transformation you were hoping for. It's also important to recognise that if you start with a BMI over 50 and achieve expected weight loss, you are still likely to have a BMI over 35 (that is, you will remain technically obese).[35]

Your *ideal weight* is taken as the weight that would give you a BMI of 25 (that is, the top end of the healthy weight range). Take a moment now to calculate your post-surgery weight goal at a realistic range of 40–70 per cent excess weight depending on the surgical procedure. You can use the BMI calculator at www.nhs.uk/tools to work out your ideal weight.

People tend to lose rather more with the gastric bypass and less with the gastric band. This should give you a rough idea as to your post-surgery target weight. Is it enough for you? Remembering that most patients will be left significantly overweight after surgery, will you feel dissatisfied if you can't lose more weight than this?

It's quite possible of course that you know someone who has achieved more than 70 per cent EWL following surgery. The average

---

Calculating your post-surgery weight

Current weight:...kg
Ideal weight (BMI 25):..kg
Current minus *ideal* weight (excess weight):............kg
Excess weight divided by 100 then × 40: ....kg = 40% excess weight
Current weight minus 40% excess weight:..............kg = **target weight at 40% EWL**
Excess weight divided by 100 then × 60: ....kg = 60% excess weight
Current weight minus 60% excess weight = ...kg = **target weight at 60% EWL**
Excess weight divided by 100 then × 70: ....kg = 70% excess weight
Current weight minus 70% excess weight = ...kg = **target weight at 70% EWL**

Your expected weight after surgery, depending on the type of surgery and your ability to maintain the changes to your diet and physical activity levels, is therefore between............. (with 40% EWL) and .... (with 70% EWL).

weight loss reported in research papers is worked out by adding together the weight loss of each individual and then dividing by the number of people in the study, so there are people who achieve more than 70 per cent EWL and you might be one of those people. But equally within that group there are people who lose significantly less than 70 per cent of their excess weight and you could be one of those as well! You can only make a balanced decision about the pros and cons of surgery if you accept a realistic weight loss. If you are having weight loss surgery for health reasons you can be confident that this level of weight loss offers major health benefits.

Preparing for surgery

There are many things you can do to prepare you for surgery, changes that, if you are able to 'get them under your belt' before going through the upheaval of surgery, could help reduce surgery risks, achieve the best level of weight loss and minimise the risk of complications. Don't wait until after surgery to think about these things, establish them as habits before surgery and you can give yourself a head start.

Change the way you eat and shop

- Start planning all meals. Keep a weekly or monthly meal planner and use this for your grocery shopping to reduce the risk of temptation purchases.
- Have three regular meals each day to prevent you from getting hungry and overeating.
- Give yourself small portions on a small plate. On average people eat 92 per cent of any food they serve themselves[37] so the more you serve up the more you'll eat. Changing from a 12-inch plate to a 10-inch plate allows people to eat 22 per cent less.[38]
- Practise eating slowly, chewing each mouthful well. Put your cutlery down between mouthfuls.
- Stop eating when you feel satisfied rather than full.
- Reduce distractions, like television or computer games, during meals so you can concentrate on the food.

Start exercising

However little or much you can manage, try to introduce some regular physical activity in your routine. Some of you may already be doing regular exercise, swimming or going to the gym, but for those who feel very uncertain about their fitness levels, walking is the easiest, safest and most convenient way to get more active.

Walking has been described as the perfect exercise. Increasing daily walking is a safe and effective way to start a physical activity routine; it gets you out of the house, helps manage stress and offers good flexibility in timing and location. Using a pedometer to measure the number of steps you take allows you to monitor your activity levels, check out your progress, set activity goals and boost your motivation. Pedometers are inexpensive and simple to use; you attach it to your belt and it counts each step you take. Most people are able to manage a gradual increase in daily steps even if health problems prevent more vigorous exercise.

You may be surprised by how many steps you take as you go about your normal activities, but you are likely to need to gradually increase daily steps. For healthy adults under 5,000 daily steps represents a sedentary lifestyle; 5,000–7,500 a low active lifestyle; 7,500–10,000 a moderately active lifestyle; and more than 10,000 steps an active lifestyle. Ten thousand steps a day may not be realistic for people with health problems or older people, but any increase in activity will have health benefits (as well as using up calories) and a pedometer provides you with feedback on your achievements, as you to move from the sedentary range to the low active, or the low active to the moderately active range.[39]

Go along to a support group

Many bariatric services run their own support groups and encourage potential patients to attend. It's an important opportunity to hear people's experiences of weight loss surgery and you can get answers to the questions you feel too shy to ask the surgeon. Having been through the surgery and experienced for themselves the challenges and successes, these patients are able to give you a different perspective from the clinical team. As well as hospital groups there are also support groups organised by the patient organisations, such as BOSPA and WLSinfo. You can find details of these organisations in Chapter 11.

> [The support group] was very helpful, I spoke to another lady who was only 4 months post op and she told me from personal recent experience what I could expect to happen pre and post op. I felt reassured.
>
> K, gastric bypass

Stop smoking

Giving up smoking is rarely easy, but this is a good time to try for a number of reasons:

- You will be fitter for general anaesthetic. Giving up smoking before surgery will reduce your risk of death and post-surgical complications, such as ulcers.
- It may help your motivation if you 'piggy back' giving up smoking on the back of a general move to be fitter and healthier.
- Finally, if the fear of weight gain has put you off giving up smoking before, you know that this will be dealt with by surgery. Your GP can talk you through the various ways you can be supported to quit.

Start a food diary

A food diary is one of the most important tools for observing and changing your eating habits. The more you understand your eating habits and triggers for overeating, the better prepared you'll be in making the changes necessary to successfully lose weight with surgery.

Keeping a food diary before surgery allows you to identify vulnerable situations or settings that tempt you to overeat or set off a binge. Once you know your high risk emotional or social situations you can work on strategies for coping with these. The ideas in the next chapter on looking after yourself emotionally may help with this.

Monitoring your food intake before and after surgery[40] can:

- Help you make changes to your eating.
- Increase your understanding of your behaviour, allowing you to identify patterns of behaviour or thinking that need to be moderated.
- Enhance your sense of control.
- Allow you to monitor your progress.

As well as supporting your pre-surgery preparation and allowing you to develop new eating habits, keeping a food diary demonstrates your commitment to the bariatric process. Some services ask you to show motivation by losing some weight before surgery and keeping a food diary will assist with this. Most importantly there is evidence that continuing to monitor your eating and drinking in the months and years after surgery leads to a better weight loss outcome.[41]

An example of a completed food diary is shown in Table 5.2. It's important to fill in the diary throughout the day rather than waiting until the evening as you are likely to forget details. Be as honest and accurate as you can; remember that the diary is for you and there is little value in being less than truthful. Though this may be painful, as you make changes you'll be able to see the positive steps you've made. Like most new habits, the benefits from keeping a food diary increase the longer you persist with it. What feels like a chore when you begin can, if you keep it up consistently for a number of weeks, become an automatic part of your routine.

Table 5.2 Example of a food diary

Date: 12th May **Day:** Thursday

Time	Food	Drink	Where? Who with?	Thoughts and feelings
8.00	2 slices toast with jam, then made another slice of toast and ate it over the sink	cup of tea, 2 sugar	kitchen	breakfast... felt hungry and had extra slice of toast, worried it's going to be a bad day
10.15	crisps	diet coke	lounge	feeling bored and alone
12.00	2 ham sandwiches... about 10 mins later had slice cake and low fat yogurt	water; tea	kitchen	lunch... know I ate too much but just feeling hungry today, also bored – stuck indoors all day
3.20	2 digestive biscuits	tea	standing up in kitchen	had these when kids got back from school, didn't even think about it
5.00	slice of bread and butter	diet coke	lounge	preparing kids' lunch boxes
7.00	shepherd's pie, mash potato, peas and cauliflower (large portion)	water	kitchen	dinner
10.30	trifle, chocolate and more crisps	2 cups tea	lounge	upset about bad day, hate how I look and worried about my health, eating makes me feel better for a while then just feel worse

When completing your food diary (you can use a small notebook that you keep in your bag or briefcase) write down the time and place where you eat, who you are with (our family and friends often influence our eating habits), what you eat/drink and, vitally, information about the situation and your thoughts and feelings at the time. This last column will provide you with essential data about social and emotional risk factors.

Some people are concerned that if they make these changes to their eating and exercise habits, they could lose weight and fall below the NICE criteria for surgery. In reality this is highly unlikely (unless you are at the very bottom end of the BMI criteria) and it is certainly a poor reason not to make these important changes. Other people say that if they could change the way they eat and exercise, they would have done it by now and wouldn't need weight loss surgery in the first place. While understandable, again this is not a good reason to avoid preparation. This thinking comes from a belief (consciously acknowledged or not) that the surgery is magical and will make these changes easy. The surgery does, of course, help you establish some control over your eating, but ultimately it is down to you to change your eating and exercise habits to produce weight loss. If you feel that you really have no capacity to make these changes (even with the motivation of surgery to bolster your attempts) you may need to question your ability to cope with weight loss surgery.

Useful information

Support with relationship issues

Relate offers relationships counselling, sex therapy and family therapy. ⚐ www.relate.org.uk ☎ 0300 100 1234.

Support for people affected by domestic violence

Refuge supports women and children affected by domestic violence. ⚐ www.refuge.org.uk ☎ 0808 2000 247.
The Men's Advice Line supports men affected by domestic violence. ⚐ www.mensadviceline.org.uk ☎ 0808 8010 327.

Support with alcohol and drug dependency

Alcoholics Anonymous (AA) offers support to people who have an alcohol abuse problem. ⚐ www.alcoholics-anonymous.org.uk ☎ 0845 769 7555.
Al-Anon supports people whose lives are affected by other people's drinking. ⚐ www.al-anonuk.org.uk ☎ 020 7403 0888.
UK Narcotics Anonymous offers support to people who have a drug problem and addicts in recovery. ⚐ www.ukna.org ☎ 0300 999 1212.

Looking after your emotional well-being

You may be wondering why a chapter about emotional well-being is sitting here in the middle of this book and what that has to do with weight loss surgery. There are three reasons why now is a good time to consider how you look after yourself emotionally and work towards developing new emotional management or self-caring skills: (i) surgery is stressful; (ii) you may have a long-standing habit of emotional eating; and (iii) surgery is an opportunity to make important changes in your life.

Surgery is stressful

The process of weight loss surgery is stressful, as is all major surgery. The difference between weight loss surgery and more standard operations is that the surgeon only does part of the job. If you have your appendix removed, a coronary artery bypass or a hernia repair, you just have to trust to the skills of your surgeon. If he/she does the job well, and you avoid the misfortune of getting an infection while in hospital, you are likely to come out the other end feeling better, less worried about your health and more able to get on with your life. With the exception of a caesarean section, there is no other common surgical procedure that requires you to make such changes to your lifestyle after the event.

As you travel through the weight loss surgery journey, your coping skills will be tested repeatedly. You will have to deal with a long assessment, living with the uncertainty of the outcome. If accepted for surgery you may be asked to demonstrate motivation by losing weight, giving up smoking, cutting down your alcohol intake and increasing exercise. You will need to follow a demanding pre-surgery diet and cope with the anxiety of your forthcoming operation date. And then the difficult part begins. The change to your eating habits and lifestyle required by weight loss surgery places huge demands on you and those supporting you. For many people this transition phase feels stressful and some patients feel emotionally vulnerable or overwhelmed. Throughout this process you will need to call upon your emotional and social resources to manage stress levels and establish a new and positive lifestyle.

You may have a long-standing habit of emotional eating

In the last chapter you had an opportunity to reflect on your personal relationship with food, whether you have binge episodes or overeat in response to upset, anger, boredom or simple availability of food. You learnt about using a food diary to record your eating, to gain insight into triggers for uncontrolled eating. For those who have identified emotional triggers, learning to cope with difficult feelings will be central to the success of surgery. Weight loss depends on your ability to manage your eating behaviour and avoid episodes of uncontrolled eating; patients who are not able to do this are far less likely to show good weight loss.

Surgery is an opportunity to make important changes in your life

Many of the patients I see describe intense feelings of guilt and shame. They feel bad about their 'failure' to control their weight, despair about their appearance and worry that they've let their family down. This pervasive sense of being *wrong* or inadequate can colour your emotional experience, making you vulnerable to feeling anxious and low, affecting your coping capacity and behaviour.

People often see weight loss surgery as a stepping stone to making a number of positive changes in their life, be it engaging in regular exercise, becoming more assertive, working to improve relationships, building a more satisfying career or developing better self-esteem. Of course the surgery will not do all of this for you; there is nothing magical in the surgeon's knife that will change overnight the person you are or your life circumstances. However, you may be able to use the motivation and confidence that surgery offers to build new skills to help you achieve your aims.

In this chapter we will discuss psychological techniques for managing stress, relieving distress and communicating effectively with others. Compassionate mind training and mindfulness skills are a good way of starting to look after your emotional well-being. You will learn about the reasons you can feel overwhelmed by painful emotions and why you may seek out food to suppress difficult feelings. You will have an opportunity to try new skills aimed at helping you become more able to accept and tolerate unsettling feelings, eat mindfully, relax your body and become kinder to yourself. You will be able to identify unhelpful beliefs that block open communication with friends and family and develop your assertiveness skills. We will also see why it's important to maintain an exercise routine for your emotional and physical health and there are some tips on how to manage stress levels day-to-day. At each stage there are practical exercises to introduce you to these new skills.

Of the approaches covered in this chapter, none are perfect for dealing with all of life's struggles and neither will they suit everyone. The main purpose of this chapter is to encourage you to spend time thinking about your emotional needs and how you will nurture your emotional health in the coming months. Bear in mind that all of the techniques considered in this chapter are *skills* – that is, they require time, patience and practice to conquer. If you find it tough to work on these skills alone, you may want to find a therapist or other helper to support you and there is information about how to find a suitably qualified therapist in Chapter 11.

Looking after . . . your emotional well-being

Why do I feel bad so much of the time?

Do you ever feel you are too harsh on yourself? Do your friends ever tell you to be kinder to yourself – to worry less about other people and a little more about your needs? Do you ever feel overwhelmed by feelings of anxiety, anger or shame, that you're just not 'good enough' in some way? Compassionate mind training[1] helps people develop a non-judgemental acceptance of their emotional experience, allowing people to be more able to understand and tolerate their emotional reactions. The skills and exercises covered in this section may be particularly important if you have a history of binge episodes, which often represent an attempt to suppress feelings of anxiety, anger or shame.

So why do we often feel overwhelmed by painful emotions and why is it so hard to let go of them? You can think of yourself as having two brains; one is the 'old brain' that deals with primitive drives, your basic survival needs. The *new brain* on the other hand has evolved an amazing capacity to think, reason, imagine and create. Compassionate mind training is based on the assumption, backed by research, that emotions are part of our *old brains* and have been hard-wired into us though evolution to protect us from threat. So anxiety, anger, sadness and frustration arise, largely out of our control, when we are faced with difficult or threatening events. These feelings are uncomfortable because they act as an alarm, informing us of a threat and the need to act to manage the threat – just like pain is an alarm to tell us that we've damaged our body. These emotions are part of a *threat-protection system*; they direct us to recognise and deal with a threat; they urge us to fight back, run away or submit. In other words they were designed to help us survive and there is no point in trying to wish them away.

The capacity of our 'new brain' to reflect, imagine, judge and deliberate, while allowing us to strive and achieve great things, can also be pulled into the services of the old brain when we experience a rush of emotion, causing our thinking to get stuck on the perceived threat; focusing our thinking on the problems causing us distress. This process is called rumination. As you get caught up in ruminating on the threat (maybe a thoughtless comment from a friend or an upcoming job interview) the angrier or more anxious you feel. Paul Gilbert (2009)[1] describes the experience of feeling caught up in strong painful emotions as like being held by a powerful magnet, however much you try to pull your thoughts away they are dragged back. We give meaning to events and to our internal experiences, such as 'I am unlovable' or 'That was unjust, I need to get them back', which intensify the unpleasant emotion.

We experience *emotional learning*, where strong emotions generated by events in the past are re-experienced in their full intensity when you are faced with an event that mirrors the original. And it doesn't require that something happens in the external world; if you are frequently self-critical, your mind and body will respond in the same way as if you were being criticised by someone else and you will feel chronically stressed and unhappy. At these times, you may become so overwhelmed by the wave of emotion that it shuts down your ability to think about helpful ways of coping, leaving you feeling helpless and hopeless. These threat emotions can make you react automatically to a situation – by becoming aggressive, submissive, avoidant or withdrawn – before you've had a chance to think it through.

As well as the threat-protection system, we also carry an *incentive-seeking system*, concerned with striving for success and achievement. The excited feeling associated with success is mediated by a neu-rotransmitter in our brain called dopamine – the same chemical involved in the 'reward' provided by highly palatable food[2] or drugs.[3] This system generates pleasurable excitement if you succeed in achieving your goal, but can also leave you wanting more and ultimately dissatisfied. This drive system is very different from the sense of well-being that comes from feeling safe and content.

Compassionate mind training is about learning to step back from the twin forces of threat-avoidance and success-drive. By becoming more observant of these events and more compassionate in your responses to yourself and others, you can begin to use your *new brain* abilities to experience positive emotions. As much of what happens in your mind is *not your fault* (as it was hard-wired long before you were born), you can stop blaming yourself for how you feel or react to events.

It emphasises the human capacity for love, attachment and joy and reflects our need for the support and kindness of others. Positive relationships with others allow us to feel safe and content. It is part of the human condition, evolved over the millennia, that we seek the approval of others and feel damaged by criticism or rejection. A third system, the *soothing-contentment system* allows you to feel safe and at peace. Unlike the drive *for more* generated by the dopamine system, this soothing, calm system is thought to be mediated by the release of the *love hormone*, oxytocin, when you feel loved and safe.[4] The compassionate mind training approach believes that we can use our capacity for calm and kindness to help soften and manage painful feelings such as shame, anger and fear. This is not a process that can occur overnight; if you have often felt threatened or anxious, your brain is very familiar with that pattern, restricting your capacity to be open to other more helpful patterns. However, stimulating the soothing-contentment system by practising compassionate mind exercises, strengthens your compassionate self and allows this voice to be heard even when your angry or anxious self is working hard to dominate. Compassion offers a balance to the frightened threat-protection system and the achievement-oriented, 'wanting more' drive-incentive system.

Compassion reflects an effort to be sensitive to your thoughts and feelings and emotionally open to your own and other people's suffering. This requires that you train yourself to *attend* to your internal experiences and to be open and curious about your experience. Instead of trying to suppress feelings (have you ever used food to do this?), you can learn to be curious about your thoughts and feelings, to *tolerate* and *accept* them in a non-judging way as they occur and then to use this compassionate attention to help guide your thinking and behaviour. So compassion can be seen as a willingness to respond openly and kindly to your suffering and the suffering of others.

Accepting and tolerating painful emotions

In order to learn to be open, curious and compassionate towards yourself and others, you need to observe and be familiar with the way your mind and attention works. One of the central skills in achieving this is mindfulness, a technique developed from the ancient tradition of Eastern meditation. Developed by Jon Kabat-Zinn[5] into a programme called mindfulness-based stress reduction, it has been shown to be beneficial when used within a range of therapeutic approaches including dialectical behaviour therapy, acceptance and commitment therapy, mindfulness-based cognitive therapy and compassionate mind training – known collectively as the *third wave* cognitive-behavioural therapies.[6]

Mindfulness is a technique that focuses on attending to the present moment without judging your experience. Human beings are, by our nature, constantly trying to make sense of our world. We spend our lives judging and assessing ourselves and our experiences. We label events and sensations as good or bad, easy or hard, acceptable or unacceptable, right or wrong, happy or sad, creating a gap between how we think things should be and how they actually are; a gap that is filled with longing, discontentment, frustration and anxiety. We also see this stretching into the future, as if the way things are now are the way they will always be.

Mindfulness has been defined as 'the awareness that arises from paying attention on purpose, in the present moment, non-judgmentally, to things as they are'.[7] By calmly observing your own reactions, without panic and without feeling compelled to act, you can shift from the *doing* domain – trying to solve problems, achieve a goal or make yourself different or better – to the *being* domain where you can 'disengage the autopilot' and stop trying to force the world to be a certain way.

When trying out any of the following exercises, make sure that you are feeling reasonably calm, warm and safe. It's difficult to learn these new skills if you are feeling particularly stressed or worried. Just as you wouldn't set out on your first driving lesson on a wet and stormy night, you will give yourself the best chance with these exercises if you don't make your first attempt when you are feeling emotionally stormy.

The first exercise is not a relaxation exercise, but rather an opportunity to focus your attention on the current moment. By keeping awareness of your attention, you know when it drifts off. In particular you can notice when your attention has been captured by an emotion or you are distracted by thoughts of other things. It is important that you experience yourself becoming distracted, as it is only through this that you can understand how your attention works and develop the skill of remaining in the moment. So becoming distracted frequently during the exercise is not a problem and does not mean that you are 'doing something wrong' or that you will 'never be able to do this mindfulness thing' – it is an opportunity to learn. So when you find your mind wandering – thinking about the shopping or that difficult encounter you had with a colleague or whether this exercise will make you feel better – simply notice the distraction and gently re-focus your attention.

This exercise in mindful attention is not about the *result* – there is no right way to feel or experience it and no particular expectation that you should feel relaxed during or after the exercise. The importance of the exercise lies in the process of noticing when your attention wanders and softly bringing it back to the task. Some people find the experience of focusing on their breath uncomfortable or even anxiety provoking. Again this is fine and does not mean that you will be unable to develop

Soothing rhythm breathing

This first exercise is a mindfulness practice using a focus on your breathing. Attending to your breathing may feel strange or uncomfortable at first. You may experience judging and critical thoughts. You do not need to worry about whether you are doing it right; however it is feeling for you is the way it's meant to feel. Simply acknowledge the distracting thoughts and bring your attention softly back to your breathing.

Sitting comfortably, place both feet flat on the floor and rest your hands on your legs. Allow your face to feel soft. Gently focus on your breathing. Allow the air to come down into the bottom of your lungs and feel your ribs move as you breathe in and out.

Just notice your breathing and breathe a little faster or a little slower until you find a breathing pattern that seems for you to be a soothing, comforting rhythm. You may find that your breathing is slightly slower and deeper than normal. If you can, keep the in and out breaths smooth and even. Spend 30 seconds or so just focusing on your breathing. You may prefer to focus on the rise and fall of your diaphragm as you breathe in and out or the sensation of air moving through your nostrils. Just focus on that for 30 seconds.

You may notice that your mind has wandered. This is fine. Notice the thoughts that occur to you and bring your attention gently back to an awareness of your breathing. The mind is unruly; the more you practise this soothing breathing exercise and the longer you extend it, the more you will notice how much your mind shifts from one thing to another. This is all very normal and expected. You are not trying to force your mind to clear itself of thoughts; just allow yourself to notice when your mind wanders, and then with kindness and gentleness bring your attention back to focus on your breathing.

Now gently turn your attention to your body, sensing your weight resting on the chair, feeling the floor beneath your feet . . . Allowing yourself to feel held and supported . . . resting in the present moment . . . Sensing the flow of air into and out of your body. Observing your experience without a need to change anything . . . just allowing things to be as they are.

When you are ready, slowly open your eyes and bring yourself back to the present moment. You may want to have a stretch and take a deep breath before you continue with your day.

(Adapted from Gilbert 2009)[1]

mindfulness skills. In the exercise above, rather than attending to your breathing you may want to focus instead on a held object that offers you a sense of calm or peacefulness, bringing your awareness to the sensation of feeling the object in your hands.

Mindful eating

Setting aside time for these exercises regularly, learning the skill of noticing distractions and bringing the attention back, allows for the mind to become more still, less liable to jump around. But mindfulness is not intended to be used only while sitting in a quiet room. The exercise on the next page is an introduction to a mindful activity, in this case eating a raisin. As you practise you will gradually feel more able to approach all activities in your everyday life, including washing the dishes or driving, with mindfulness.

In mindfulness-based therapy, raisins are often used in this exercise, but of course it could equally well be an orange or an apple. After surgery, you will need to eat slowly and thoughtfully, avoiding certain foods. Bringing mindfulness to your eating can help this process; asking yourself if you are really hungry, whether you are using food as a distraction from other feelings, allowing yourself to feel the sensations of hunger and fullness and truly savouring the taste of your food will help you in your efforts to eat slowly and thoughtfully. Try practising mindful eating for just the first one or two bites of each meal, gradually building up the skill so eating can become a real pleasure in your life rather than a way to shut off other experiences. Avoid other distractions during the meal – turn off the TV and the computer – and focus on truly enjoying the smell, the tastes and texture of the food in your mouth as you chew.

Relaxing the mind and body

The body scan exercise described on p. 89 is more directly concerned with producing feelings of calm relaxation, to release feelings of stress and tension and to enable open, kind and accepting contact with your body in the present moment, using the breath to guide awareness to each part of the body. While stress and tension are a bodily response designed to allow you to deal with threat, the body also needs to learn that it can let go of this tension. To get the most benefit, it is recommended that you practise the body scan daily, ideally using a guided meditation CD.

You may be feeling a little overwhelmed by the idea of these new skills and I guess you could already be telling yourself that you simply don't have the time. Ideally you would set aside some time each day to practise the mindfulness and compassionate thinking exercises. By doing them regularly you are retraining your mind to be more able to

The raisin exercise

This exercise is frequently used as an introduction to mindfulness, allowing you to experience the difference between ordinary doing and mindful awareness. By spending a few minutes on this exercise, you can begin to sense the intensity of experience you can access if you focus your full and non-judgemental attention on the simple act of eating. As with all mindfulness exercises, when distracting thoughts surface – and of course they often will – notice them and gently bring your attention back to the task.

Take a raisin and hold it in the palm of your hand. Imagine you have never seen a raisin before and take time to really see it, your eyes exploring every aspect of its appearance; its colour, the way the light falls on the folds and ridges.

Explore the texture of the raisin; how does it feel between your fingers?

Bring the raisin up to your nose and allow yourself to experience any aroma. Notice any changes that occur in your body; does your mouth respond to the thought of eating the raisin by producing saliva? Do you notice any sensations in your stomach?

Bring the raisin slowly up to your mouth, attending to the movement of your body and the feel of your muscles as you raise your arm. Place the raisin in your mouth without chewing. Allow it to rest on your tongue, exploring the sensation of having it in your mouth and noticing how the texture feels against your tongue.

Think about chewing the raisin and attend to the feeling of anticipation. Roll the raisin around with your tongue. Consciously chew the raisin once or twice, fully attending to the sensation of biting through the raisin and the taste and texture in your mouth. With each chew notice the changing sensations.

Try to detect the intention to swallow before you swallow, notice consciously how your mouth prepares to swallow and when you feel ready allow yourself to swallow, trying to remain aware of the sense of the raisin moving down towards your stomach, attending to how you feel after completing this exercise.

(Adapted from Williams *et al*.2007)[7]

remain focused and calm. If you have found the idea of being kinder to yourself (and to others) quite scary, you are not alone in this. If you struggle with feelings of anxiety or anger or have an entrenched habit of self-criticism, you may find it difficult to believe that you can

Simple body scan relaxation

Find a space where you can lie comfortably, where you are warm and unlikely to be disturbed. Relax on your back with your arms by your side and your palms facing upwards. Allow your eyes to close and focus on your breathing until you find a rhythm that is most comfortable and soothing for you. When you are ready, bring your awareness to the physical sensations of your body and as you breathe out allow yourself to sink a little deeper onto the bed or mat.

Focus on your legs and notice any sensations such as warmth or cold, heaviness or numbness. As you breathe in become aware of any tension in your legs. Imagine the breath passing down through your body and into your legs and on the out breath coming back up through your body and out through the nose. When you are ready, as you breathe out imagine all the tension in your legs flowing out of your body.

Now focus on your body, from your shoulders down to your stomach, again breathing into this part of your body and, as you breathe out, imagining the tension leaving your body and flowing away. Be aware of your kindness to your body as you let go of the tension.

Now focus on your fingers, wrists, arms and shoulders. Being aware of any tension in this part of your body as you breathe in . . . and as you breathe out releasing the tension and letting it go.

Now focus your attention on your head, neck and forehead. Being aware of any tension you hold in your head and neck. Imagine how your body would like to release this tension. Breathing into this part of your body and as you breathe out, imagining all the tension flowing away with your breath.

Now focus on your whole body. Each time you breathe out focus on the word 'relax' or 'calm'. Imagine your body becoming more relaxed and feeling heavier on the surface you are lying on. Continue to breathe in this way, enjoying the feeling of relaxation.

When you are ready, end the exercise by taking a deeper breath, moving your body a little. Notice how grateful your body can feel, being given permission to let go of tension. When you are ready, stand up slowly and continue with your day.

(Adapted from Gilbert 2009)[1]

access a feeling of calm and safety. You may feel that you don't deserve kindness from yourself or others; that being kind to yourself would make you selfish; or you may worry about other people's reactions to these new ideas. These are understandable reactions (which you can notice with curiosity and kindness). To begin with you may need to take it on trust that compassionate mind training will, if you persevere, 'exercise' your compassion skills (just as you would expect to train up your fitness before taking on a physical challenge) and allow you to feel comfortable with these new experiences. It is important to take it at your own pace and leave exercises for a while if they make you feel troubled.

If you have found this introduction to the ideas of mindfulness and compassionate mind training interesting, you can read more about them in Paul Gilbert's *The Compassionate Mind*[1] and *The Mindful Way through Depression* by Mark Williams *et al.*[7] which includes a guided meditation CD with body scan and mindful breathing exercises narrated by Jon Kabat-Zinn. Guided meditations by Dr Kristin Neff, a leading researcher in self-compassion, are available to download free from www.self-compassion.org.

Looking after . . . your relationships and social support

Why do I struggle to communicate openly with friends and family?

> Be who you are and say what you feel, because those who mind
> don't matter and those who matter don't mind. [8]

Being able to draw on others for help and support is an essential part of the changes you must make after weight loss surgery. Requesting practical and emotional support, saying 'no' to unrealistic requests and being able to express your thoughts and feelings openly will be critical tools in the weeks and months after surgery as you make adjustments in all aspects of your life. Social support, a sense of being loved and valued by others, is known to have enormous benefits in terms of better health and improved emotional well-being.[9]

Even if you are surrounded by warm, loving friends and family – and I certainly hope you are – developing more assertive communication may still be challenging, especially if you are used to putting your needs after those of your loved ones and are unpractised in telling others about your wants and needs. Others of you may be in a place in your life where you feel isolated from other people and that there is no one you can call on for help. You may be in a relationship that is unsatisfying, controlling or abusive. These situations will bring very particular challenges to coping with weight loss surgery and you may need to talk to your bariatric team or GP about how you can access additional support.

Where children grow up with critical and demanding parents, they are vulnerable to internalising these parental criticisms and becoming sensitised to being hurt or rejected by others. To compensate they may develop perfectionistic standards – 'I must never show anger', 'I must never make mistakes or show weakness' – to avoid anticipated criticism and rejection from others. Instead of being seen as a source of help or caring support, other people are perceived as a source of threat.[10] Many of the people I see in clinic talk about a constant striving to be 'good', to do their best in order to escape from relentless internal criticism. As they fear that others will reject them 'if they see the real me', they have great difficulty in expressing their wishes and opinions. They are blocked by fears that their requests will be refused or that they will be seen as selfish and demanding. Others worry that asking for help will make them appear weak and vulnerable, unable to trust that others won't take advantage. Do you recognise yourself in these descriptions? Do you find yourself pushing people away and becoming aggressive in difficult situations or do you submit to other people's wishes? Do you expect others to understand instinctively what you want or need, telling yourself that if your family and friends 'really' cared for you, they should know? Ultimately all of these reactions are likely to generate feelings of frustration or leave you with a sense of being alone, overlooked and uncared for.

Above we spoke about developing skills in compassion as a way of accepting and tolerating difficult emotions rather than getting stuck in self-criticism. As you use develop your compassionate self, are less judging of your thoughts, feelings and reactions and more able to be open to feelings of compassion towards others, you may find yourself being more emotionally open. Sometimes being compassionate means dealing with challenging situations, talking candidly with others, and this is where assertiveness comes in.

Blocks to self-expression

Assertion has been defined as 'the flexible pursuit of having our preferences met, our opinions voiced, our emotions and beliefs honestly communicated in an appropriate way at the relevant time';[11] in other words, being open about your own wants and needs while respecting those of others. It is not about aggressively demanding that your needs are met at the expense of others nor is it passively giving in to the wishes of others.

Aggressive or passive communication habits arise out of unhelpful beliefs about yourself, the world and other people.[11] These beliefs inhibit open and clear communication of personal needs, wants and opinions due to a fear of the potential consequences. Most non-assertive communication represents an attempt to avoid uncomfortable situations or feelings, but in the long term has a more negative impact. It can be helpful to start by thinking about the unhelpful beliefs that impact on the way you communicate with others. Use the exercise in Table 6.1 below to identify your communication style. You may want to write down your own assertive response rather than use the ones I've suggested.

Respecting your own needs and opinions

Assertiveness emphasises the importance of caring for yourself, respecting your own needs and opinions and being able to communicate these simply and directly to other people in a way that neither undermines your wishes and opinions (as in passive communication) nor attempts to bulldoze over their wishes (with aggressive communication).

Windy Dryden and Daniel Constantinou (2004)[11] outlined eight principles central to assertive self-care:

1. Say 'no' when it's appropriate and accept that others may do so also.
2. Express your emotions, opinions and beliefs when appropriate and accept that others may do so too.
3. Acknowledge that you will make mistakes and accept yourself for making them. Others will also make mistakes.
4. Be yourself without believing that you have to be different for someone else's benefit. Accept that others can be themselves too.
5. Allow yourself to change your mind even if this is inconvenient for others, and accept that others may also change their mind.
6. Accept that you can make decisions others find illogical, but do not necessarily have to offer an explanation. Accept that this also applies to others.
7. Do not take responsibility for finding solutions to others' problems and accept that others will not take responsibility for yours.
8. Feel comfortable about stating your ignorance or lack of interest and accept also that this applies to others.

You will see that all these principles apply equally to yourself and those around you. They emphasise that no individual is worth more than any other, that all people are unique with their own thoughts, beliefs, feelings and preferences. The foundation of close and meaningful relationships is based on your right to look after your needs and wishes, recognising your individual worth, while acknowledging the unique needs and preferences of others around you.

Table 6.1 Identifying unhelpful communication beliefs

Unhelpful belief	What are you avoiding?	Communication and behaviour	Assertive belief
If I don't follow other people's wishes and expectations they won't like me.	Anxiety. Disapproval from others.	Passive communication: dismissing own wants and needs, self-criticism. Putting other people first.	No one can be liked by everyone. If I try, I take on too much and lose my sense of what I want and need. It may not be nice to feel that someone disapproves of me but I can cope.
I need to get my own way.	Feeling powerless or frustrated. Fear of others 'getting one over'.	Aggressive communication: demanding, insisting on being right, not listening to the other's point of view. Being denigrating of other people's opinions.	Being aggressive may get me what I want, but at a high price. It makes it difficult for me to feel close to people and I often feel the need to be on the look-out. I feel guilty after I've upset someone I care about. I may not always get my own way if I communicate assertively, but I can cope with a compromise sometimes.
If I say no to other people's requests, I am being selfish and will let other people down.	Discomfort of self-criticism. Fear of rejection by others.	Passive. Unable to refuse requests. Putting other people first. Using up physical, emotional and financial resources in meeting others' expectations.	I can look after my own needs without being selfish. Relationships need to be based on give and take. I have the right to say no to others.
If I disagree with other people they will reject me.	Anxiety. Fear of rejection.	Passive communication. Not communicating opinions openly. Suppressing sense of self. Agreeing with others.	I have a right to express openly my thoughts and opinions. It is important to recognise my own individuality and this helps me feel more confident. Rejection is very upsetting, but I can tolerate it.
If I'm open about my feelings with others, they will be upset.	Guilt. Discomfort.	Passive. Reluctant to express your emotions. Feeling guilty and emotionally responsible for the other person.	I have a right to express my feelings. Talking about how I feel with someone may be uncomfortable for them, but I have no reason to think that they can't cope with it.
Other people should know what I want/need.	Discomfort of talking openly. Fear of being refused.	Passive and aggressive – refusing to talk about feelings because others should know instinctively. Getting angry and frustrated when they get it wrong.	It would be great if people always knew what I wanted, but it's unrealistic to expect people to be mind readers. If I tell people what I want directly I have a better chance of getting it.

Communicating effectively

So how do you start communicating assertively? There are some characteristics of assertive communication which offer the best chance of having your preferences met or a suitable compromise found. If you watch someone who is communicating effectively and assertively you will tend to see and hear:

- The regular use of *I* statements, such as 'I feel . . .', 'I would like . . .' or 'I do not agree'. *I* statements are clear and direct. They require you to take responsibility for what you are saying.
- A firm, calm tone of voice and steady speech. Assertive communication does not need you to shout your opinions at the other person, but does require that you be heard. Keeping your voice steady and at an appropriate volume, without too many pauses, helps to communicate that you want your comments to be taken seriously.
- An open, relaxed body posture. Staying at the same level as the person you're talking to so you can communicate as equals.
- The use of open questions – that is questions that can't be answered with a *yes* or *no*. Good examples of open questions are: 'How do you feel about . . .?' 'Where would you like to go from here . . .?' or 'What would you like to change about . . .?'
- The use of checking and clarifying statements. These are used to make sure you have understood the person correctly; 'So you feel that we should . . .', 'I think you're saying . . ., is that right? ' and 'You say you feel upset about . . .'.
- Acceptance of the other person's comments if you accept their validity, such as: 'I know that sometimes I don't stick to time as well as I should.' If you don't agree, you can still indicate that you've heard their comment: 'You feel that I don't stick to time. I believe that usually I'm good at this.'
- Statements to bring the discussion back to the main point: 'You feel that I don't stick to time as you would like and we need to talk about that another time. I would like to focus on my request that we go out together more regularly.'
- Offers of compromise based on an understanding of both people's point of view. Assertiveness is founded on the flexibility to look for a solution that may not be your ideal, but gets both you and the other person closer to where they'd like to be.
- Clarification of the agreement: 'So we have agreed that . . .'.

In order to feel confident using these skills you may have to do some preparation beforehand. Reflect on the situation you are approaching and consider what emotions are coming up for you. Are you feeling worried or angry in anticipation of the conversation?

Identify the belief linked to that emotion and create a more helpful assertive statement. Think carefully about what point you are trying to make and plan a compromise in advance; if you can think through a *win–win* situation that suits both of you, it is more likely to be accepted and offer a good outcome. Rehearse in your mind (or in front of a mirror) what you will say and how you'll say it. Think about timing; your discussion may need some time and you will want to make sure neither of you is too hurried or tired to give it their attention. After a difficult communication spend a little time debriefing. Did you get your point across? Did you become aggressive or passive during the communication? How did the other person respond to your comments or request? Did you come out with an agreed compromise? Is there anything you should remember for next time about what worked or didn't work?

As with any new skill, developing assertiveness skills can feel challenging. It may generate feelings of anxiety or vulnerability. People around you, familiar as they are to your old style of communication, may not respond as positively as you would hope initially. So start out small and build up. You will need to think more consciously about what and how you communicate, so begin your practice with situations where you feel reasonably confident. Being assertive with acquaintances or strangers tends to be easier than raising emotionally loaded issues with close friends and family.

> If someone else is cooking it might be difficult to eat what they have made – but now I put myself first and don't eat it and don't worry about upsetting them or even pleasing them.
>
> C, gastric bypass

Draw up a list of situations in which you'd like to communicate more effectively and write them out in order of order of difficulty, from easiest to most challenging, as in Table 6.2. Set a goal to be assertive in the easiest condition, observe how it feels and the reactions you get from others. Use your mindfulness skills to calm unruly emotions. Once you feel confident being assertive in relatively *safe* circumstances, try the next step and so on.

Remember that assertive communication is not a magical solution to all problematic situations and just as you have the right to be open about your wants and opinions, so does the other person!

Looking after ... your physical well-being

No doubt you have been told many times in your life by doctors, friends and even strangers that you should exercise more. 'If you just did more and ate less you wouldn't be in this situation' is a refrain commonly

Table 6.2 Assertiveness practice

Joanna F

Difficulty	Achieved	Task
1	✓	Take broken shoes back to shop. Ask for refund.
2	✓	Ask neighbour for a small favour, e.g. to get a bit of shopping.
3	✓	Ask Paul to look after the children on Saturday morning so I can go to the gym.
4	✓	Being honest about my opinions in a conversation about politics.
5		Approach someone I don't know well in the school playground and start a conversation.
6		Talk to friends about my feelings.
7		Tell Sophie that I felt hurt when she missed my birthday.
8		Talk to Paul about learning mindfulness skills. Ask him to support me . . . join in?
9		Talk to my boss about going on to part-time hours.
10		Talk to mum about <u>not</u> commenting on my weight.

heard by people who struggle with their weight. Yet many overweight and obese people have had negative experiences of trying to exercise; swimming can make you feel self-conscious, the gym seems full of sleek bodies and jogging is uncomfortable.

There are, however, many good reasons for finding a way to incorporate exercise into your life. Regular physical exercise has proven benefits including improved cardiovascular fitness, greater strength and stamina, better muscle tone, more energy and faster weight loss – all of which are going to help your overall sense of well-being. Importantly, there is also good evidence that a regular exercise routine reduces symptoms of depression and anxiety.[12,13] One study of identical twins showed that the twin who engaged in regular vigorous exercise showed higher levels of optimism, sense of control and better mood than their non-exercising twin, despite sharing the same genetic inheritance.[14] The benefits of physical exercise on emotional well-being are likely to be a complex combination of psychological and neurophysiological factors. Exercise provides an opportunity to develop a more positive self-image, a sense of mastery and is a distraction from worries, while increased production of certain brain chemicals is also thought to be related to the psychological benefits of exercise.[13]

Finding the right exercise routine

One of the difficulties of exercising when overweight or obese is finding a suitable level to start at and then sticking at it. You are certainly not alone if you have difficulty maintaining motivation; two-thirds of adults in the UK fail to meet government recommended exercise levels.[15] One issue is that people want exercise to feel reasonably easy and to have immediate payback. If you think exercise shouldn't involve getting hot, sweaty and out of breath your internal critic is likely to kick in when your experience doesn't match your expectations. If you are telling yourself 'I'll never be fit, there's no point trying' or that 'Nobody wants to see me in a swimming costume', it will make it a lot harder to persevere. However, if you can gently challenge these thoughts and tolerate the feelings of anxiety and hopelessness they generate, you will be more able to maintain your exercise routine, despite it feeling tough sometimes.

Generally a combination of aerobic exercise (exercise that gets you slightly breathless) and resistance training is most effective in reducing symptoms of depression and anxiety.[16] The general advice is to aim for 150 minutes of moderate to vigorous physical activity a week and this can include *lifestyle activities* like gardening, dancing, walking the dog and so on. By including relatively short bursts (at least 10 minutes at a time) of physical activity into your daily routine, you can build up your active minutes towards the 150-minute total. If that sounds more that you can manage, remember that you'll be working up to this over the months as you lose weight.

If you are new to exercising it's important that you build up your physical condition gradually. For example, you could start by walking an extra 10 minutes every other day for a few weeks before slowly increasing the time and speed of your walking. As you feel more confident, work up to 20–30 minutes of moderate intensity exercise three or four times a week and expect to keep that up for a couple of months to experience the long-term advantages, though some benefits such as feeling calmer and revitalised are more immediate.[17] Gentler exercises, such as yoga and tai chi, have also been shown to improve depression and anxiety.[16]

Start an activity diary of *formal* exercise and active daily activities (such as walking the dog, gardening or dancing) to keep up motivation and monitor progress. You could also record your mood in this diary to assess the emotional benefits. Remember, focus on making *some* change and don't worry so much about the level initially. Set yourself realistic, achievable goals to build your confidence. There is more information about increasing physical activity in Chapter 8.

Looking after . . . your stress levels

There exists a mountain of research on stress and the impact of stress on emotional and physical health. There is no one agreed definition of stress, but it can be thought of as a physiological and psychological response to a perceived threat requiring the mobilisation of physiological and psychological resources. We feel stressed if the perceived threat outweighs our available resources.[18] Chapter 2 discussed how cortisol, the 'stress hormone', can impact on weight gain and stress is also known to affect our mood and decision-making ability.

There are two broad categories of stress management strategies; those that focus on resolving the problem and those that aim to moderate your emotional reaction to a stress. The first category, problem-focused coping, would include problem-solving, prioritising demands or communicating with others around difficult issues. These strategies work best where there is something that can be done to control or manage the stress. The other category, emotion-focused coping strategies, include such things as mindfulness, imagery techniques or seeking emotional support from others and are most useful when there is nothing that can be done to control a stress. So, for example, in preparing for a challenging job interview you might use problem-focused strategies, information gathering, question preparation, rehearsal and so on, to give yourself the best chance of doing well. After the interview there is no longer anything you can do to affect the outcome so emotion-focused strategies would be more helpful in dealing with any nervousness or worry.

The ability to respond with *self-kindness* to difficult emotions and situations, using the compassion skills we spoke about earlier, will help you balance competing life demands and regulate your reaction to stressful events[19] but there are a number of other daily strategies you can use to help manage stress levels and keep yourself on an even keel. The different strategies are divided into approaches that help you actively manage stress in your life, those that are concerned with managing your emotional response to stresses, and finally those aimed at building up your emotional resources or nurturing yourself.

The kind of stress management strategy needed in any particular situation is not always as clear; the art in knowing how best to tackle stress is often in knowing what problems you can actively control and which you can't. It is frustrating, as well as a waste of energy, to problem-solve a state of affairs that is out of your control, but if you don't actively tackle situations you *can* control you are missing an opportunity to resolve the difficulty.

Strategies for actively managing sources of stress

1. Identify your priorities. With all tasks decide whether they are *urgent or non-urgent* and *important or not important*. Make sure that you prioritise important, urgent tasks and don't get too tied up in jobs that feel urgent, but aren't actually very important. It is also essential to make time for tasks that are *important*, but *not*

urgent; tasks that are easy to put off, but which could make a big difference to your quality of life, like practising your mindfulness exercises, looking into that new job you want, training in a new skill or spending time with friends.

2. Know what you value in life. In order to prioritise well, according to what is truly important to you, spend some time thinking about those aspects of your life that you value most. Think about what you value in terms of *loving relationships, work* and *leisure* and how you would like these aspects of your life to look if you could create your ideal world. Are you exactly where you would like to be in terms of your loving relationships, feeling close to others and able to communicate that closeness? In terms of your work, what would your work life look like right now in the world you created? How would work make you feel? What would you be doing? Again think about how near or far you are from your real work values. Finally in the domain of leisure, what would you be doing in your free time? Do you have an opportunity to do things that you find pleasurable? In your ideal world what would you be doing? Now, identify the three main barriers between you and the life that you value. What are the obstacles? Do you persevere in trying to overcome these obstacles? You may be able to make only small changes and it may take you outside your comfort zone, but try to make a commitment to taking a step towards your valued future.[20] If you encounter problems on the way, look at the problem-solving strategy below.

3. Solve problems actively. When faced with a problem, do an assessment of the best solutions. Write down all the solutions you can think of and rate each potential solution on the basis of how helpful it is (that is, how likely is it to resolve the problem) on a scale of 0–5 (with 0 being the least helpful and 5 being the most helpful) and on how difficult it would be to carry out (again on a scale of 1 least difficult to 5 most difficult). Using this assessment, decide on your preferred strategy, the one that you think is realistic but has the best chance of dealing with the situation. Follow through with this strategy and monitor the outcome. If it works, that's great. If not go back to your original list and try the next most helpful, most realistic solution.

4. Be aware of demands on your time and emotional resources. You may need to practise saying 'no' to requests that are more than you can handle. If you are uncertain whether you are able to meet someone's request, ask for time to think about it. Try not to allow yourself to feel rushed by people; rushing tends to lead to mistakes and more stress. Use soothing-rhythm breathing to calm your body and mind and focus on the task at hand.

Strategies for coping with the emotional impact of stress

1. Identify your stressful situations. Make a list of events that leave you feeling emotionally drained or anxious. When they arise, use these situations as a trigger to practise your mindfulness exercises.
2. Use imagery to deal with anxiety before a big event. Making use of soothing-rhythm breathing to calm your mind, run through the event, picturing yourself coping despite anxiety or misgivings. If you need to give a speech at a wedding or do a presentation at work, you can improve your performance by mentally rehearsing your talk a number of times. By approaching tasks or challenges in a mindful way – being open and curious, rather than critical, of your feelings and reactions – you can minimise *catastrophising* thinking which generates intense anxiety and panic.
3. Let go of past events. If you feel upset about a poor decision you made in the past it may help to write it down. Writing down your recollections of a difficult event and sealing it in an envelope can help to weaken the memory and reduce its emotional power. People asked to do this report a sense of psychological closure.[21]

Strategies for building up your emotional resources

1. Focus on small pleasures. For example, if you like to go for a walk in the country or by the sea you should pay attention to the experience of this pleasure. Notice the feeling of the air on your face and the sounds and smells around you. Notice the sensations of your moving muscles as you walk along, perhaps experiencing a satisfying tiredness as you get near the end of the walk and anticipate the pleasure of relaxing at home.
2. Do an act of kindness for another person.
3. Write about a time when you feel you were at your best and reflect on the personal strengths displayed in the story. You could also use the 'personal strengths questionnaire' available at www.authen tichappiness.org. When you've identified your personal strengths try to use them in new and different ways each day for one week. This exercise has been shown to increase happiness and reduce symptoms of depression.[22]
4. Count your blessings. Keeping a daily *gratitude* journal, regularly writing down the things in your life that you feel grateful for, has been shown to help people feel more optimistic, have greater life satisfaction, feel more likely to achieve life goals, be more energetic and experience fewer physical symptoms than people asked to record neutral life events.[23]
5. Get enough sleep. Compared with people who sleep happily through the night, those people who sleep less than five hours a night are

five times more vulnerable to developing high blood pressure.[24] Lack of sleep also leads to higher ghrelin levels and increased appetite.[25]

Summary

- Adapting to life after weight loss surgery is a challenge; it calls on all your practical, emotional and social resources. However, it is also an opportunity to make positive changes in your life.
- The experience of painful emotions is part of the human experience. Powerful emotions arise from our 'old brains' and alert us to danger. Emotions such as fear and anger act as a 'threat-protection' system and, because they were designed to help us survive, they can overwhelm other more positive feelings.
- It helps to recognise that you are a human being who (like the rest of us) sometimes feels overwhelmed with emotions and may sometimes struggle with situations and make unhelpful choices. Use this awareness to be kinder to yourself.
- Practising mindfulness daily can help you accept and tolerate difficult emotions. The practice of mindful eating may help manage emotional eating. Remember to remove distractions including the television and computer during mealtimes and focus your attention on the tastes and textures of the food.
- You will need considerable support from others while adapting to life after weight loss surgery. Think about what obstacles prevent you from communicating openly with others. Build on your assertiveness skills by drawing up a list of challenging situations and tackling them one at a time.
- Establish an exercise routine based on your existing fitness level. It's better to do a little every day than to knock yourself out once a week. Recognise that for everyone building up physical fitness is a slow and challenging process and no one expects you to be out running marathons (unless that's your dream).
- There are two broad approaches to managing stressful situations. Problem-focused coping, like problem-solving, prioritising and assertive communication, are most useful in situations where you have some control. Emotion-focused strategies, including mindfulness and relaxation, are best when there is little that you can do to change a situation. Other strategies, such as making use of your personal strengths and keeping a gratitude journal, can be used to increase positive emotions and build up your emotional resources.
- There are a lot of new ideas and skills in this chapter and you may be left feeling a little overwhelmed. It would be unrealistic to make all the changes immediately, so you might want to think about making one change at a time and gradually incorporating them into

your life. Remember that all skills become easier the more you practise. Keep a diary of the changes you make and monitor your mood. It will motivate you to continue your efforts and remind you of how far you have come.

- While many patients who go through weight loss surgery feel better, reporting fewer symptoms of depression and improved quality of life,[26,27] a small proportion of people experience a worsening of their emotional health (see Chapter 10). If at any stage you feel that you're struggling to cope or experiencing raised anxiety or distress it is essential that you quickly access help and support through your GP or mental health team.

Useful information

Support with mental health problems

Samaritans provides emotional support to people in distress 24 hours a day. ⌨ www.samaritans.org ☎ 08457 90 90 90.

Mind offers information and advice to people with mental health problems and can guide people towards local services. ⌨ www.mind.org.uk ☎ 0845 766 0163.

7

Weight loss surgery:
the facts and figures

This chapter covers the information you need to understand the different weight loss procedures and their risks and benefits. While the gastric band and the gastric bypass are the most commonly used procedures on offer, your surgeon may also talk to you about the sleeve gastrectomy, intragastric balloon or biliopancreatic diversion/duodenal switch (BPD/DS). In this chapter there is information about the surgical process, the benefits and potential difficulties or complications for each of these procedures as well as preparation for surgery, what to expect when you wake up from the operation and follow-up appointments.

In the UK at least 7,000 bariatric procedures were performed in 2009 and 2010;[1] just over half were gastric bypass, a third were gastric band and the others were made up of sleeve gastrectomy, gastric balloon and other less common procedures, such as duodenal switch. Worldwide, the commonest procedure is the gastric bypass[2] though the gastric band and sleeve gastrectomy are being increasingly used in the USA. The sleeve gastrectomy is a newer procedure and so there is less information about its long-term benefits and complications.

The decision [about the choice of procedure] is made, depending on what type of eater you are and what type of food you eat, because if you are a crisp and chocolate eater you can cheat the band, because you can chew these up so that it slides past the band, and you do not get a good weight loss. However, with the bypass, you cannot cheat, because, if you over-stuff, it gets stuck, which is very painful, or if you eat something with too much sugar or fat, you can suffer from the dumping syndrome, which makes you feel sick, shaky and dizzy, I don't much fancy any of those, so I behave with my food, and as I eat properly and slowly, I do not suffer ill effects and the weight loss is significant.

K, gastric bypass

Before surgery

Two weeks before surgery

Most surgeons expect you to follow a special pre-surgery diet for one or two weeks before surgery. The purpose of this diet is to shrink the liver by reducing its stores of glycogen and water. The surgeon has to move the liver to access the stomach during weight loss surgery, so by reducing the size of the liver before surgery you minimise the risk of surgical complications.

> [The pre-surgery diet] was a very strict, low carb, low protein and low fat diet. Everything had to be weighed and quantities were very small. I stuck to it religiously – I was terrified that if I did not I wouldn't lose any weight and . . . be sent home again on op day.
>
> K, gastric bypass

> [Before the pre-surgery diet] I expected to go on a binge and so did my husband, but I didn't. I so wanted the op I didn't want to jeopardise my chances . . . This felt like my last chance to get my life back.
>
> J, sleeve gastrectomy

The details of the pre-surgery diet depend on your bariatric team, but it will be low in carbohydrates, sugar and fat. Some services recommend a 'milk only' diet while others offer a range of diet options. The dietitian will give you detailed information about what you can and can't eat at this stage.

Examples of *daily* pre-surgery dietary restrictions include:

- five pints of semi-skimmed milk *OR*
- four cans of low calorie diet soup and four low fat, low sugar yoghurts *OR*
- four low fat low sugar yoghurts plus 1 litre (2 pints) of semi-skimmed milk *OR*
- a low calorie, low fat, sugar and carbohydrate diet, including lean meat or fish with small amounts of carbohydrates and vegetables.

You will need to ensure that you take plenty of fluids, especially in warm weather. You are allowed water, tea and coffee (with no sugar) and small amounts of diet drinks. You may also be advised to take a vitamin supplement.

> I had to do the milk diet for 1 week pre op, because my BMI was less than 45, otherwise it would be 2 weeks. I did find it quite hard because my husband ate normally during that week and the smell

of his food was torture. To escape this and the risk of cheating I. . . had a long bath. I did not cheat once.

K, gastric bypass

I found the [pre-surgery diet] confusing and stressful [however] I lost 11lb in those two weeks.

N, gastric bypass

Many people find this diet difficult and you may feel irritable or unwell initially, but it's important that you stick to it carefully. Just one large 'last supper' of high fat or starchy foods could undo all your efforts. It has been known for surgeons to refuse to proceed with the operation if the liver is too large so making the surgical risks too great. If you have struggled to follow strict diets in the past beyond a few days or if there are particular reasons why you may not cope with the pre-surgery diet it is important to talk to the dietitian so you can be offered additional support.

My motivation to keep on the diet was the threat of the surgeon not performing the op due to the liver being too big.

J, sleeve gastrectomy

As I am a compulsive eater anyway I just carried on eating for Britain.

J, gastric bypass

You may also be asked to walk regularly and carry out breathing exercises to reduce the risks of complications after surgery. Most surgeons will expect you to have given up smoking before surgery.

A few weeks before the operation, you will attend a pre-admission assessment clinic. This is an opportunity to check that you are prepared for your admission, treatment and discharge home. You may need routine investigations such as blood tests, ECG (to record your heart function) or a chest x-ray to check your fitness for surgery. An anaesthetist will also see you at this appointment. If you take blood-thinning medication (such as warfarin or aspirin) or have any allergies to medication you need to inform the staff at the pre-admission assessment. You also need to inform the team if you have any particular anxieties about injections or general anaesthetic.

Twenty-four hours before your operation

You are not allowed to have anything to eat or drink after midnight the night before your operation. If you need to take medicines, you should take them early on the morning of your operation with a small sip of water. If you are on medication for diabetes you will be given advice from the bariatric team as to when to stop your medication. If you are being admitted on the day of the operation you will need to organise your things to take in to hospital; nightclothes and toiletries, and also any medication and your continuous positive airway pressure (CPAP) machine if you use one.

On the day of your operation

You will be admitted to the ward and your temperature, blood pressure, respiration rate, height, weight and urine will be taken. You may be measured for special stockings (sometimes known as 'TEDS') to prevent blood clots forming in your legs following surgery and started on anti-coagulant (blood-thinning) injections to help minimise this risk. You will need to remove all make-up, nail varnish, jewellery, body piercings and dentures.

You can expect to have access to suitable equipment, such as bariatric beds and chairs and pressure-relieving mattresses.[3] The surgeon will explain the procedure to you before asking you to sign a consent form to ensure that you understand the potential risks of the operation.

Almost all bariatric surgery is now carried out with laparoscopic (keyhole) surgery, where the operation is performed through small cuts, using video cameras and special surgical equipment. The advantages of laparoscopic surgery are less scarring, not as much pain and quicker recovery. If the surgeon believes it will reduce risk, for example by making the procedure quicker, they may convert to open surgery.

How does weight loss surgery work?

The various bariatric procedures have typically been categorised broadly as *restrictive* or *malabsorptive*. It was originally thought that bariatric surgery allowed you to lose weight either by simply limiting how much you could eat, that is with the gastric band and sleeve gastrectomy, or by a combination of restriction and a reduction in the absorption of calories, as with the gastric bypass or BPD/DS.

We now know that while all procedures have an element of restriction this is not sufficient to explain the dramatic effects they produce and the mechanisms producing weight loss are more complex than initially thought. With the gastric band, physical restriction of food intake is of relatively minor impact but rather it seems, by ways not yet fully understood, to increase satiety.[4] While before it was felt that both the gastric bypass and BPD/DS prevented the absorption of calories to produce weight loss, it is now clear that the main effect is likely to be through changes in gut hormones that allow the brain to regulate hunger and satiety (though the BPD/DS does also cause malabsorption of calories). Both sleeve gastrectomy and BPD/DS have been shown to result in decreased levels of the hunger hormone, ghrelin.[5] Though the most common procedure, the mechanisms of weight loss in gastric bypass are perhaps the least well understood, but research continues to look at the impact of this surgery on the balance of 'keep eating' hormones and 'stop eating' hormones.[6]

Laparoscopic adjustable gastric band (LAGB)

The gastric band (Figure 7.1) is one of the most frequently used bariatric procedures. It involves fitting a silicone band around the

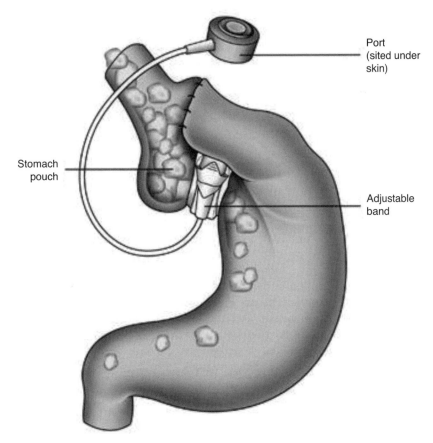

Figure 7.1 Gastric band. Reproduced with permission from the Imperial College Healthcare NHS Trust

upper part of your stomach. Once the gastric band is in place, the stomach pouch above the band is divided from the main part of the stomach by a narrow channel. The band may be stitched in place to prevent slippage. The band is fitted using keyhole (laparoscopic) surgery under general anaesthetic.

The gastric band is termed a 'restrictive' procedure, though it seems to work primarily by reducing the amount of food you eat by increasing satiety (full) signals rather than physical restriction. Once the food has moved through to the lower part of the stomach it is digested normally.

The band usually needs to be adjusted a number of times to regulate the level of restriction. The band is tightened by injecting a saline solution though a metal port that sits under the skin on the abdomen. This is called a 'band fill' and takes approximately 30 minutes. The band can be loosened by drawing saline out through the port. The tighter the band, the smaller the channel, the slower food passes through and the more restricted you are in how much you can eat. You do not usually have your first band fill until a number of weeks after surgery.

Success with the band is judged by rate of weight loss (with an expectation of weight loss of ½ –1kg per week), restriction in eating, and satiety (fullness) with meals, together with an absence of excessive vomiting. Initially you will have to return to see the bariatric team every few months to see how you are getting on and to have further band fills if you are feeling that your food intake is not restricted (or is too restricted) or you are not losing weight.

You will need to follow a liquid diet initially, moving on to a soft diet of pureed food after a couple of weeks, then more normal foods after a month or two. You may experience some difficulty in swallowing, which is an expected sign of food restriction, but most people are able to tolerate a varied diet once the band has had a chance to settle. You need to be careful with certain foods, such as bread, pasta, rice, red meat and some fibrous fruits and vegetables as they can cause bloating or blockage. Many patients feel that being unable to eat certain foods, particularly bread and red meat, is the most troublesome problem after surgery.[7] Fizzy drinks are not recommended as they can cause complications. The bariatric dietitian will give you detailed instructions on suitable foods post-surgery and there is more information in Chapter 8. As with all bariatric procedures the band is most effective if you maintain a regular exercise routine.

What are the benefits?

The gastric band allows you to feel full quicker and for longer and so supports you in having a much lower calorie diet. The band is adjustable, so the size of the opening between the pouch and the main part of the stomach can be varied to regulate weight loss. The gastric band offers an average weight loss of around 40 per cent of your *excess weight* by one year post-surgery and 50 per cent excess weight by two years[1,8] and some gastric band patients continue to lose weight for as long as three years after surgery. That means if you weigh 120kg and your healthy weight is 70kg, the band should help you lose around 25kg. However, there is a lot of variability in how much weight people lose with the band; when patients are followed up over a number of years, less than half maintained over 50 per cent of excess weight loss.[9] By ten years after surgery, around a quarter of gastric band patients will have returned to within 5 per cent of their pre-surgery weight.[10]

The band is less invasive and easier to reverse than other weight loss procedures. It is involves a shorter stay in hospital (many patients being able to be treated as day patients[11]) and more rapid recovery compared to gastric bypass. You are able to return to normal activities of daily living, including work, sooner than with the more invasive procedures.

Between five and seven out of ten patients show an improvement or resolution of diabetes/insulin resistance[12,13] and dyslipidaemia. Almost half of patients will experience a resolution of high blood pressure and two-thirds will show improvement or resolution of sleep apnoea.[12] Unlike the gastric bypass, improvement of the components of metabolic syndrome (insulin resistance, hypertension and hyperlipidaemia) following gastric banding is dependent solely on weight loss. Gastric band patients also report enhanced general health, social functioning and energy levels.

What are the disadvantages and risks?

As with all surgery, the gastric band carries risks. Around 2 in every 100 patients will need to be re-admitted to hospital in the weeks following surgery, and on average one of these will need a further operation to correct a problem.[14] Some of the complications are serious and require further surgery, such as erosion and band slippage. In the years following gastric band, some research studies have found that 1 in 20 gastric band patients need some kind of further surgery or treatment to manage complications, mainly slippage, erosion or problems with the port.[7] A further 5 per cent experienced minor complications, such as iron deficiency, urinary tract infection or breathing difficulties shortly after surgery.

The band may require a number of adjustments to find the right point of restriction to ensure that your eating is limited and you have a sense of fullness when you eat small amounts of food, but not overly restricted. For some people it is difficult to find the perfect level and it can take some trial and error and repeated band fills.

Some people with the gastric band are able to tolerate only a limited range of foods or find they regularly vomit after meals, with around 20 per cent of patients being moderately or severely bothered by this. Frequent vomiting should not be treated as normal and expected; you need to check you are following the dietary guidelines and are taking care to chew all food slowly and carefully. Continued excessive vomiting can increase the risk of complications, including slippage and pouch dilation, so you need to talk to your bariatric team if it persists. There is more information about the complications of gastric band in Chapter 10.

The band can become obstructed if you eat certain foods, such as bread, pasta, red meat or fibrous fruits and vegetables. If you are unable to vomit up the food, you need to go to hospital to have the band loosened to allow the food to pass through into your stomach. Some patients suffer from reflux (heart burn) and bloating.

Around 15–20 in every 100 band patients do not achieve the level of weight loss that would be hoped for and expected. A small number of gastric band patients experience weight regain to above their pre-surgery weight.[9] If you do not show good weight loss with the band you may be offered a further bariatric procedure, usually gastric bypass, depending on the availability of funding.

Sleeve gastrectomy

The sleeve gastrectomy (Figure 7.2) is a more recent procedure than the band or bypass. Patients having sleeve gastrectomy tend to have a higher BMI than gastric band patients. The sleeve gastrectomy was originally developed as a first stage procedure for patients felt to be too high risk for gastric bypass or biliopancreatic diversion, before surgeons realised that it offered good weight loss in its own right. It is now often used as a stand-alone bariatric surgery, though you may still be offered a sleeve as an interim procedure before having gastric bypass if you have great deal of excess weight or health problems that make surgery more complicated. Conversion to gastric bypass following a sleeve gastrectomy carries higher risks of complications than a primary gastric bypass.[15]

The sleeve gastrectomy divides your stomach vertically in a line using medical staples, converting the stomach into a long, thin tube (shaped rather like a banana) and reducing the size of your stomach by about three-quarters. The staple line is then cut through and the main part of the stomach removed. The procedure cannot be reversed.

The sleeve gastrectomy causes you to eat less because you feel less hungry and experience a feeling of fullness and satisfaction with much less food. Unlike the gastric bypass, the food still passes through the whole stomach before entering the small intestine. People who have

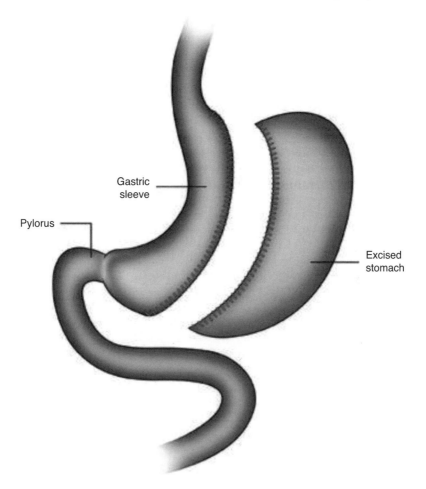

Gastric
sleeve

Pylorus

Excised
stomach

Figure 7.2 Sleeve gastrectomy. Reproduced with permission from the Imperial College
Healthcare NHS Trust

the sleeve tend to want to eat less, are more able to stick to three small
meals a day and so lose weight.

You will need to avoid heavy lifting for a time but most people are
able to return to work after a few weeks. You will be on a liquid-only,
then pureed and soft food diet for a number of weeks after surgery,
before slowly introducing soft normal food. After about six weeks you
can return to a more normal diet.

What are the benefits?

The sleeve gastrectomy offers an average weight loss of around
55 per cent[1] to 60 per cent of your *excess weight*.[16] That means if you

weigh 150kg and your ideal weight is 75kg, the sleeve should help you lose around 41kg.

The sleeve allows you to feel full quicker and for longer. Many patients who have sleeve gastrectomy show an improvement or resolution of diabetes/insulin resistance,[17] high blood pressure, sleep apnoea and dyslipidaemia.[3] Many patients also report better emotional and physical well-being.[18] There is relatively little long-term information about outcome with laparoscopic sleeve gastrectomy, compared to the band and bypass, as it is a newer procedure.

What are the disadvantages and risks?

The sleeve gastrectomy offers a greater degree of weight loss compared to the gastric band, but also carries higher risks. Complications can include leaks through the staple line, infection, bleeding, strictures and pulmonary embolism (a blood clot in the lung). The length of hospital stay is longer for the sleeve gastrectomy than the gastric band.

About three to five in every 100 sleeve gastrectomy patients will need to be re-admitted to hospital in the weeks following surgery and on average three of these will need a further operation to correct a problem, such as leakage from the staple line.[1,14] Up to 15 per cent of sleeve patients show complications, inadequate weight loss or weight regain in the first year after surgery.[18] You may develop gallstones as the result of rapid weight loss which could require an operation to remove your gallbladder and you will need to take medication to reduce stomach acid each day for a few months. The sleeve gastrectomy is not reversible.

Roux-en-Y gastric bypass (RYGB)

With a gastric bypass (Figure 7.3) the stomach is stapled to make a small pouch. The staple line is cut through so the pouch is no longer attached to the main part of the stomach. The surgeon divides the small intestine approximately 75–150cm down from the top of your small intestine and attaches this to the stomach pouch. The connection of the intestine to the stomach pouch is called an anastomosis. As the main area of the stomach is stapled off, food no longer goes through this, but rather passes straight from the oesophagus into the stomach pouch and then to the small intestine. The end of the small intestine that is still connected to your stomach is then attached to the small intestine joined to the stomach pouch, to allow digestive juices to pass through into the small intestine.

The gastric bypass was originally thought to restrict food intake and alter the absorption of calories, but these are no longer believed to be the main mechanisms of weight loss (though gastric bypass does

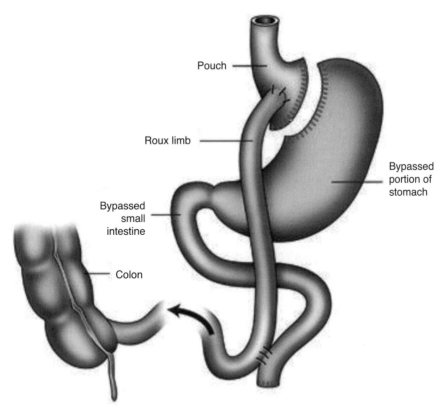

Pouch

Roux limb

Bypassed portion of stomach

Bypassed small intestine

Colon

Figure 7.3 Roux-en-Y gastric bypass. Reproduced with permission from the Imperial College Healthcare NHS Trust

affect absorption of certain nutrients). It certainly helps you eat less; many patients feel much less hungry after bypass surgery, are satisfied with much smaller portions and less interested in food.

You will need to follow a liquid diet initially, after a couple of weeks moving on to a diet of pureed food, gradually trying a soft diet over the following months. This soft diet reduces pressure on the gastric pouch and allows time to heal. After about six to eight weeks you will be able to return to a more normal healthy diet. The dietitian will provide you with detailed information about suitable foods for the early months after surgery and you will need to attend hospital for regular follow-up checks. You will need to avoid heavy lifting for six weeks or so, but most people are able to return to work after a few weeks.

There is considerable variation between patients in what foods gastric bypass patients can tolerate, with some people having difficulty with bread, meat and pasta. If you consume foods high in fat, sugar and starch (e.g. chocolate, ice-cream), you may start to feel unwell; this is known as *dumping syndrome* and causes dizziness, palpitations, anxiety, stomach cramps and diarrhoea. It is due to a reaction in the small intestine to sugar that has not been processed through the stomach. While this side effect can be very unpleasant, it does tend to reinforce the need to avoid certain unhealthy foods and so can support the change to a healthy diet.

> I once made myself unwell . . . I was brought some sugar free marmalade, which was made for diabetics so should have been fine, but I got the dumping syndrome with it. I had awful diarrhoea and the shakes in my body. I felt very sick, so I chucked it in the bin, and have not eaten it again.
>
> K, gastric bypass

The bypass is potentially reversible, for example in the case of unremitting dumping syndrome, alcohol dependency or excessive weight loss, but reversal is associated with rapid weight regain. Conversion to a sleeve gastrectomy is also possible but carries increased risk of complications such as staple line leaks. Reversal or conversion procedures should only be carried out at specialist centres.

What are the benefits?

The gastric bypass offers an average weight loss of 60–70 per cent of your *excess weight*[1,12] with patients often showing some weight regain in the longer term. This equates to about 30–35 per cent of your body weight at one year after gastric bypass, though by ten years the average maintained weight loss is 25 per cent of your pre-surgery weight.[10]

With an average loss of 65 per cent excess weight, if you weigh 150kg and your ideal weight is 75kg, the bypass should help you lose around 50kg. People with a pre-surgery BMI over 50 show more weight loss, but because of their higher starting weight are still likely to be significantly overweight. The bypass tends to produce faster weight loss than the gastric band and you would expect to reach your target weight about 18 months after surgery.

Patients don't generally feel hungry in the same way after gastric bypass, as the procedure causes changes to the gut hormones that help regulate appetite.[6] Some patients describe a loss of interest in food as it no longer has the same reward value for them.

Around 84 per cent (more than eight out of ten) gastric bypass patients show an improvement or resolution of diabetes or insulin resistance[19] often with normalisation of blood sugars levels occurring soon after surgery as a result of changes in gut hormones. Most patients will also see improvements in other comorbidities, such as hypertension, hyperlipidaemia, sleep apnoea and non-alcoholic fatty liver disease, as well as better general health, social functioning and energy levels.

What are the disadvantages and risks?

Just over six in every hundred gastric bypass patients will need to be re-admitted to hospital in the weeks following surgery, and five of these will need a further operation to correct a serious problem, such as bleeding, leakage or obstruction.[14] A further 15 per cent of patients will experience early minor complications, such as dehydration, urinary tract infection, wound infection or diarrhoea. In the longer term around a quarter of patients (25 per cent) will have more major complications, including narrowing of the opening from the stomach to the intestine, internal hernia, ulceration of the stomach, abdominal pain or obstruction. There is more information about potential surgical and medical complications in Chapter 10.

You will need to take multivitamins and minerals daily for the rest of your life, and have regular blood tests to monitor your nutritional status. Some people experience inadequate protein absorption – which can lead to loss of muscle mass and hair loss – so gastric bypass patients need to be very careful to maintain their intake of protein by eating the protein first in any meal and may need to take protein supplements. You can develop gallstones as the result of rapid weight loss which could require an operation to remove your gallbladder (*cholecystectomy*). Gastric bypass may not be suitable if you have epilepsy as it can affect the absorption of anti-epilepsy medication.[20] The bypass is reversible but reversal surgery carries risks and can only be done through a specialist centre.

Biliopancreatic diversion/duodenal switch (BPD/DS)

The BPD/DS is less commonly used than the gastric bypass, generally only being offered to patients with a very high BMI. This procedure creates a stomach pouch about a quarter of the size of the stomach removing the remainder of the stomach, like a sleeve gastrectomy. The small intestine is then attached to the stomach pouch. The part of the intestine previously attached to your stomach joins the small intestine from the new stomach pouch at the *end* of the small intestine, leaving a much shorter digestive channel than with the gastric bypass so the absorption of food is significantly reduced. Food remains undigested and fewer calories are absorbed. As with the other procedures, PBD/DS helps you feel less hungry and satisfied with smaller portions.

The BPD/DS bypasses pancreatic and bile drainage, so absorption of fat and sugars is very limited. Patients can eat larger quantities of food than with other procedures, because the stomach pouch is bigger, and still lose weight because of reduced absorption of calories, but may experience frequent loose bowel movements and unpleasant flatulence especially if they have a diet heavy in fatty or starchy foods. This type of surgery is very technical and only partly reversible. The BPD/DS can be carried out as a second stage procedure after sleeve gastrectomy.

What are the benefits?[21]

BPD/DS can offer a very good level of weight loss; an average loss of up to 70–75 per cent of *excess weight* at 12 months and 90 per cent EWL at two years post-surgery. That means if you weigh 150kg and your ideal weight is 75kg, biliopancreatic diversion should help you lose around 55–65kg.

When you eat, you will feel full quicker and for longer. You will be restricted in how much you can eat and will feel full after a relatively small amount of food, but the stomach pouch is bigger than in gastric bypass so allowing larger portions. Almost all patients show an improvement of diabetes or insulin resistance, often with some normalisation of blood sugar levels only days following surgery. The majority of patients also show significant improvements in hypertension and hyperlipidaemia, which can be maintained up to ten years post-surgery,[22] and sleep apnoea.

You are less likely to experience dumping syndrome than gastric bypass patients, because the valve that controls food passing from the stomach to the intestine is left intact.[23]

What are the disadvantages and risks?[21]

BPD/DS is a complex procedure and so carries greater risks, particularly for patients with a pre-surgery BMI over 65. BPD/DS is not commonly used (only making up 0.1 per cent of all bariatric procedures in recent years[1]), though it can produce very substantial weight loss, as it is associated with significantly higher risks and problematic side effects which can affect patients' quality of life. Most patients are not willing to accept the side effects and complications. The BPD/DS has a mortality rate of around one in a hundred patients (1 per cent) when carried out by an experienced surgeon.[12]

Complications include bleeding or leakage through the staple line; the development of ulcers or internal hernias potentially causing block-age of the stomach pouch or intestine. Vomiting is common if you eat too much or too quickly and BPD patients experience bad smelling flat-ulence and loose stools if they continue to eat high fat and sugar foods.

Protein, vitamin and mineral deficiencies are a relatively common problem and people with BPD/DS need to work hard to ensure they maintain high levels of protein in their diet. You will need to be monitored closely for protein malnutrition, anaemia, and bone disease, take multivitamins and minerals daily and have regular blood tests to monitor your nutritional status. You are more likely to experience iron, zinc, copper, calcium, vitamin A and D and protein deficiencies than gastric bypass patients.[24] A very small number (less than one in 1,500) of BPD patients develop a serious neurological problem, known as *Wernicke's encephalopathy*, within a few months of surgery[25] and your ability to comply strictly with the multivitamin and mineral supplements is something your bariatric team will consider during assessment.

Up to 60 per cent of BPD/DS patients develop gallstones due to rapid weight loss and you may need a further operation to remove the gallbladder. To prevent the need for further surgery some surgeons remove the gallbladder during the initial procedure.[26]

Intragastric balloon

An intragastric balloon is a soft silicone balloon that is implanted in your stomach. This procedure can be done without making an incision in your abdomen; instead, the balloon is passed through your mouth and down into your stomach using an endoscope (a thin, flexible tube that is fitted with a light and a camera). The balloon is filled with a saline solution (salt water) and takes up some space in your stomach, so you do not need to eat as much as before to feel full.

This procedure is only temporary and the balloon is removed after six months. The gastric balloon may be useful if you do not meet the criteria for the other types of surgery or if the risks of undergoing surgery are too great. It is most commonly used as an interim procedure to reduce risks before going ahead with gastric bypass or sleeve gastrectomy. If you are having the balloon as a stand-alone procedure you will need to make long-term changes to your eating habits and lifestyle to prevent weight regain when the balloon is removed.[27]

What are the benefits?

Fitting the intragastric balloon is a relatively straightforward and non-invasive procedure. It is fully reversible and carries fewer risks than other procedures. The gastric balloon should make you feel full quicker so you eat less. Average weight loss is around 12 per cent of total body weight at six months.[28] That means if you weigh 150kg the intragastric balloon should help you lose around 18kg.

Depending on the amount of weight lost, an intragastric balloon can offer important health benefits, with improvements in insulin sensitivity, blood pressure and hyperlipidaemia.[27]

What are the disadvantages and risks?

Randomised controlled trials with intragastric balloon have not shown conclusively that it produces better weight loss than a standard approach to weight management[29] and most people will regain the weight they lost with the gastric balloon if they do not have further weight loss surgery.[28] The gastric balloon is intended as a short-term intervention and within the NHS is mainly used to get you down to a weight where you can have a permanent bariatric procedure with less risk.

Some patients experience stomach pain, nausea and vomiting, especially if they are unable to control their eating despite the balloon. A small proportion of patients (just under 5 per cent) are unable to tolerate the intragastric balloon and have it removed early. The balloon can cause inflammation of the lining of the stomach or oesophagus. Serious complications are unusual, but obstruction can occur if a deflated balloon passes into the intestine and this would usually require surgical removal. Gastric perforation is a rare but life-threatening complication.

Deciding on the best procedure for you[26]

The clinical team will support you in deciding which procedure is right for you depending on your preferences, weight and medical needs. Through the assessment, as they get to know you and develop a clear understanding of your needs, the team will consider the following: (i) how much weight you need to lose; (ii) your eating habits; (iii) how quickly you want or need to lose weight; (iv) your concerns about the risks of surgery; (v) history of abdominal surgery; (vi) whether you have strong teeth; and (vii) your alcohol consumption.

How much weight you need to lose

The gastric bypass and BPD/DS offer greater overall weight loss compared to the gastric band. The sleeve gastrectomy generally allows people to lose more weight than the band but somewhat less than the gastric bypass.

Your eating habits

If you consume a lot of chocolate, sweet foods and high fat foods you are less likely to have a good outcome with the gastric band as it will not restrict your consumption of soft, high calorie foods. With the gastric bypass you are likely to be discouraged from eating sugary, fatty foods because of the unpleasant side effects. If you eat relatively little a band is again unlikely to be helpful, as it works by cutting down on the amount you eat, and the gastric bypass might be a better option. Vegetarians will need to discuss options with the dietitian; with both the gastric bypass and BPD/DS you need to ensure that you get adequate protein in your diet.

How quickly you want or need to lose weight

The gastric bypass and biliopancreatic diversion offer rapid weight loss with most of the weight coming off in the first 12 months after which weight loss slows down. With the gastric band you see slower, steady weight loss over a number of years. Some people want to see their weight coming off as quickly as possible, while others prefer more gradual weight loss. Slower weight loss allows you time to adjust to your new body and self-image. If you have ever felt distressed or vulnerable after rapid weight loss though dieting (as sometimes occurs with low calorie, liquid-only diets), you may want to take this factor into account.

Your concerns about the risks of surgery

It's natural to be worried about operations and anaesthetic, but for some people this is a source of significant anxiety. If you are very fearful of surgery and don't like to stay in hospital, the gastric band may be a better option as the length of surgery and stay in hospital is generally shorter. You are also less likely to require readmission for further surgery with the band compared to the gastric bypass, but you will need to be willing to attend regular outpatient appointments for band fills.

History of abdominal surgery

If you have had a number of operations on your abdomen it may be more difficult to do the bariatric procedure through keyhole surgery and you may need open surgery.

Whether you have strong teeth

In order to cope with the gastric band, you need to be able to chew your food very carefully. If your teeth only allow you to eat soft foods, the gastric bypass or sleeve may be a better for you.

Your alcohol consumption

If you have had a problem with excessive alcohol consumption, the team may feel that the malabsorptive procedures, gastric bypass and BPD, are unsuitable because of the effect of these procedures on the way the body handles alcohol.

After surgery

After surgery you will wake up in the recovery room before being taken back to the ward or high-dependency unit. The nurses can help if you are in pain or feel sick. You may feel light-headed or sleepy after the operation due to the anaesthetic. It is also common to have a sore throat for a couple of days after having general anaesthetic, because the anaesthetist has to pass a tube down your windpipe. You will be asked to get up and move around shortly after surgery, as this will reduce the risk of complications, such as DVT (deep-vein thrombosis), and speed your recovery. You may be asked to do breathing exercises to reduce the risks of blood clots on the lungs. Your wound will have been closed with sutures (stitches) that dissolve within seven to ten days after surgery.

A catheter may be used to drain urine and to allow the nurses to monitor your urine output and this is usually removed after a couple of days. You may also need a tube to drain away any blood or fluid from your wound to prevent swelling for two or three days. A drip will be attached to a needle in your arm or neck to provide you with fluids and prevent dehydration. You will be given a supply of medication to take home with you and any medication you need after that will be prescribed by your GP.

With the gastric band you may be able to go home the same day or the next day. The hospital stay for gastric bypass, sleeve gastrectomy and biliopancreatic diversion is longer as they are more invasive and complex procedures, usually three to five days. You will need to organise someone to collect you by car on the day of discharge as you will not able to drive yourself or travel on public transport. If you have had the gastric bypass, sleeve gastrectomy or biliopancreatic diversion you will need to avoid heavy lifting, strenuous activity and driving for a number of weeks. Your team will give you information about appropriate activity and breathing exercises.

You may have some abdominal discomfort in the first week, which can be caused by your wound or the reduced size of your stomach. You can take painkillers for this if necessary, but check with the bariatric team what medication you can safely use. You may have tingling, itching or numbness sensations in your wound and these are a normal part of the healing process. If you experience a high temperature, swelling, pain, discharge or excessive redness around the wound site, you need to see your GP or go to the local accident and emergency department promptly as you may have an infection.

After surgery you will be expected to attend for regular follow-up meetings with the bariatric team to check the surgical wounds are healing well. For the gastric band you may need to have a number of band fills before you can settle at the correct level to achieve steady weight loss. The first band fill is usually six to eight weeks after surgery. Most services expect you to maintain a regular exercise programme after surgery to promote weight loss. Your exercise should be *low impact*, such as walking and swimming, at least initially so it doesn't put too much strain on your joints.

In the months after the operation, your bariatric team should continue to offer regular follow-ups to monitor progress; providing information on the appropriate diet, checking your nutritional status, advising on individualised nutritional supplements, and offering support and guidance for long-term weight loss and weight maintenance.[30] Between appointments, you need to contact your bariatric team if you encounter any difficulties, such as excessive vomiting, pain, feeling unable to swallow or a significant change in your emotional state.

Making a decision about weight loss surgery

The decision about whether or not to have weight loss surgery is a very personal one. All procedures carry medical risks and require long-term determination and motivation to offer the best results. Only you can decide whether the potential risks are outbalanced by the likely benefits as these will be personal to you.

Each procedure offers different levels of risks and benefits. The highest risk is associated with biliopancreatic diversion and the least with the gastric band. The level of risk is consistent with expected weight loss; broadly the procedures with the higher rates of complications offer greater weight loss, so biliopancreatic diversion offers greatest weight loss, followed by the gastric bypass, the sleeve gastrectomy and then the gastric band.

You should by now have enough information to consider your decision on whether or not weight loss surgery is something you want to proceed with and, if so, which procedure you'd prefer. In order to do this you need to be clear and precise about the factors affecting your decision.

To take a business analogy, all important decisions involve a trade-off and knowing what you can't achieve is as valuable as being clear about what you will pursue. How do you know which trade-offs are good business and which are losing propositions?

The *Harvard Business Review* suggests three important elements to making a decision that has both advantages and disadvantages:

- List the advantages and disadvantages and get input from other people. Get a perspective on how important each is.
- Balance short term and long term. What are you willing to give up short term for long-term gain? Can you accept the long-term losses?

- Get a sense of the support available to you. Who will support your decision, who will oppose it? Whose support can you live without and whose backing do you absolutely need?

Having read this chapter take some time to write down your personal pros and cons. Reflect on what you really want from surgery and how able you are to make the changes to your diet and lifestyle to make it a success. For each benefit or disadvantage, judge how important it is to the decision and score it on a scale of 1 to 10, where 1 means it's of little importance and 10 is of major importance. Scoring each item helps you to see which ones are the most relevant to your decision. Look at Table 7.1 to give you an idea.

Return to your list as you go through the assessment and add or change things as you learn more about weight loss surgery. Remember the tendency is to assume that the risks 'can't happen to me' as you focus on the benefits. By making the decision to have surgery you are accepting the risks and difficulties that can go with it. If you are uncertain about your decision ask your bariatric team for more time; do more research, talk to people who have had surgery and check out your ability to change your eating habits. If you decide to go ahead with surgery, keep your list of reasons; it's easy to forget 18 months down the line, after you've lost a lot of weight, what your life was like before surgery. If you feel frustrated that you haven't reached the weight you'd hoped for, it helps to look back and see the big changes in your health and emotional well-being that you've achieved.

Table 7.1 A score sheet of benefits and disadvantages

Julie – October 2010

Benefits	Score	Disadvantages	Score
Improve my diabetes	10	Worry about vomiting	9
Able to play with the kids	10	Miss my favourite foods	6
More energy/sleep better	8	Worry about how people will react	7
Improve my blood pressure	9	Planning all meals feels like chore	8
More able to go on holiday	7	Don't like exercising	6
Be able to buy nicer clothes	4	Scared of general anaesthetic	9
Be healthier in future	10	Eating everything slowly	5
Not getting out of breath	7	Eating out will be strange	3
Feel more confident	4	Lots of food I can't eat	6
Won't have to take so many tablets	5	'This is forever'	9
		Risk of complications	6

I would say to people [thinking about surgery] – do lots and lots of research into weight loss surgery, talk to other people who have had it done, think very hard about the changes to your life that you will need to make, both physical and mental changes. Be very sure this is what you want, and then go for it.

K, gastric bypass

8

'Pressing the re-set button': life after weight loss surgery

Knowing that I was going to have the surgery and my new life would be starting after that. I was getting to press the re-set button.

K, gastric bypass

In general, studies have found that weight loss surgery is associated with improved outcomes for patients with greater life expectancy, reduced reliance on medication, better quality of life, more confidence, less depression and more control over their eating. However, this experience is not universal and the road is not always smooth (as you will see in Chapter 10). Pressing the re-set button on your life, as it was described by one patient, can be a pretty scary business; everything that has been familiar to you – what you eat for dinner, how you cope with worry or upset, how others respond to you, your image in the mirror – all will be changed and uncertain. However much you want these changes, the process of adjustment can be hard work.

Some people have described the process as like being reborn[1] and there seems to be a distinct psychological process, described in a paper by psychologist Jane Ogden and her colleagues[2] that patients go through before arriving at their GP surgery to request weight loss surgery. A background of failed diets and weight cycling leads to a profound sense of lack of control over eating and weight gain. People often live for years with profound distress as their weight affects every aspect of their emotional, social and physical well-being, creating the backdrop to the desire for control over weight through surgery. The final decision to speak to their doctor is often triggered by a specific event. Already feeling powerless about their weight, the diagnosis of a weight-related illness or the loss of someone close can activate fears of disability and death; the birth of a grandchild can push a desire to participate in life more fully; a frustrated life goal, such as starting a family, shifts a general unhappiness into an urgent need to get something done. It is in this context of powerlessness, a desire to 'shift the control of their problem over to something outside themselves' (Ogden *et al.* 2006: 281)[2] that leads to patients to embark on the weight loss surgery journey.

> [Surgery] has given me a 'tool' to control my eating. I joined Weight Watchers in 1969; signed up with Dr . . . of Harley St in 1970 . . .; signed up with . . . .in 1993 and went on to put on another 6 stones; [I] did the Cambridge, the cabbage soup diet, back to Weight Watchers, joined the gym, took up yoga, took up pilates . . .
> You name it NOTHING had the effect this operation has had.
>
> J, sleeve gastrectomy

Some patients assume that surgery equals permanent weight loss without effort and believe that the surgery will magically allow them to make the necessary changes to their diet and exercise. The research clearly shows that this is not the case; patients that do best, those who lose the most weight, feel better and have improved quality of life with minimal weight regain, are those that are aware of their responsibility in maintaining these changes in the long term.

> I have spent years and years locked in a very lonely body, going downhill all the time. I hope this is my ladder to help me.
>
> J, gastric bypass

In the context of this overwhelming sense of being out of control of their weight and eating behaviour, weight loss surgery patients often feel a great feeling of new hope, describing surgery as the start of a new life, the possibility of a 'new me'.

> It was time to acknowledge that I could no longer accomplish this kind of weight loss on my own.
>
> A, gastric bypass

However, many patients find the initial aftermath of surgery stressful and disorientating; feeling fatigued, unwell or in pain, struggling to adjust to a new way of eating and finding it difficult to tolerate food.

> The second week was really tough because I felt weak and tired.
>
> N, gastric bypass

After surgery you will be required to overhaul your eating behaviour and lifestyle; these changes don't happen automatically, there's nothing in the surgeon's knife that will do all this for you. It will require motivation, determination and hard work to achieve success. The patients who do best are those who use surgery to establish healthy habits; who engage in regular exercise; set themselves goals; monitor their food intake, mood and exercise; use stress management approaches (like those in Chapter 6); manage their environment to reduce temptations to overeat; call on their social network for help and support; attend follow-up appointments; and attend a support group.[3] In this chapter we will look at the transformations you will need to make in the weeks and months after surgery as well as the strategies you can use to help you maintain these changes.

Changing your eating habits

You will be provided with detailed instructions about what and how to eat after surgery by your bariatric dietitian and it's important that you follow that advice carefully. The information below is designed to give you a broad idea of how you'll need to adjust your eating post-surgery. Immediately after surgery you will be on a liquid only diet, slowly incorporating thicker liquids, pureed and soft foods over the following months before moving on to a more regular varied diet. This gives your stomach pouch time to heal or the band to settle. Eating solid foods or overeating during these early stages can reduce the effectiveness of surgery or cause serious complications. How quickly you can move from one stage to the next will vary from person to person, but it's important to allow plenty of time for your body to adjust and you should never try to move on to the next stage more rapidly than advised by your team (usually at least two weeks at each stage). If you have problems at any stage, speak to your dietitian or nurse specialist before moving on to the next stage.

Stage 1: liquids

This is a liquid only stage. It starts immediately after surgery and lasts for about two weeks. You will normally be allowed to take small sips of water the morning after surgery. Make sure you have different drinks to ensure that you're getting adequate nutrition. You can include semi-skimmed milk; thin yoghurt; smooth soups; dilute fruit juice; drinks made from Bovril or Marmite; sugar-free squash; tea and coffee with sweetener; build-up drinks; milky drinks (with semi-skimmed milk); and sugar free jelly. Avoid fizzy drinks or sparkling water, alcohol, liquids with bits in, and high fat, high sugar drinks such as creamy milkshakes.

Drink small amounts during the day and avoid drinking past the point of feeling full. Think about having six to eight cups a day, about 100–200mls over the course of an hour, and include one pint of semi-skimmed milk and one to two glasses of dilute fruit juice each day. Even though you're only having liquids try to stick to mealtimes, sitting down to have a small yoghurt, a cup of soup or meal replacement drink at regular times. Between meals you can sip on water, squash, tea or coffee.

Stage 2: pureed food

Again you need to think about having a balanced diet as you move on to pureed foods, so include a range of foods that will provide you with the necessary vitamins and nutrients. Eating too much or drinking large quantities of fluids will cause vomiting. A poor diet can lead to loss of muscle mass, hair loss and dry skin.

Even though the food is very soft, chew all food well and allow yourself 30–45 minutes for a meal. Drinking while eating can cause food to be washed through the stomach pouch too quickly, causing you to become overly full and uncomfortable, so avoid drinking for 30 minutes before and after a meal. Continue to eat at regular times, sitting down and taking your time over the meal and stop eating as soon as you're full. Start to incorporate pureed vegetables (with the skins removed); potato and sweet potato; thin scrambled egg; chicken, fish or quorn in gravy; pureed or mashed fruit; mushy breakfast cereals; and yoghurt. Use a blender or potato masher to ensure that all foods are the consistency of porridge. Avoid skins on food, such as tomato, grapes or apple skins, sausages, and foods that are not easily chewed, like lentils, bread or toast, nuts, chickpeas and sweet corn. Continue to have semi-skimmed milk (one pint a day) and dilute fruit juice.

Stage 3: soft textured food

In this stage you can begin to introduce soft foods, but there may be a number of foods that you can't manage. You will need to chew all food thoroughly to avoid stomach pain; focus on eating slowly, listening for your body's signals of being full to prevent vomiting and discomfort.

Your meals in this stage should be made up of soft, mashed foods. Keep an eye on your diet to make sure you are taking in a range of nutrients and to avoid falling back into eating large amounts of high fat or sugary foods. In addition to the foods you have already introduced, try soft cereals, such as porridge; mashed potato; soft cooked pasta; mashed vegetables or baked beans; cottage cheese; minced chicken or fish in a sauce; dry toast; soft omelette; and tinned fruit. Have three meals a day, allowing yourself plenty of time for each meal. Serve yourself a small portion on a side plate and avoid drinking half an hour before and after eating. Avoid alcohol, which can irritate the stomach and fizzy drinks. Steer clear of fibrous foods, like red meat, celery and pineapple, and foods with skins or seeds, like tomatoes. Meat may also be difficult to tolerate, but you can try mince.

Stage 4: healthy, balanced diet

In this stage you should focus on establishing a healthy balanced diet, incorporating a wide variety of foods. This is the time when you will create the foundation for your new eating habits, so it's important to base your diet around healthy nutritious foods, rather than slipping back to old habits of relying on high calorie foods, which may feel easier to digest or more comforting. The groundwork you do now will determine the success of surgery, affecting long-term weight loss and your health.

Remember that your stomach is now much smaller than it was – imagine the size of an egg-cup – and adjust your portions accordingly. If you continue to serve yourself large portions, relying on the surgery to limit your eating, you will gradually train your new stomach to accept more food. Just a few mouthfuls taken after you feel full can, over time, lead to less restriction and weight regain. Eat slowly to reduce the risk of vomiting and to help you be aware of your hunger/ fullness levels.

> [It's difficult] going out for a meal and leaving half my food, coming from a culture where you finish everything on your plate, it took a lot to just leave food and be happy doing it.
>
> A, gastric bypass

After surgery, the protein in meals is your first priority; an adequate protein intake is necessary to prevent the loss of lean muscle mass and enhance satiety. Your meals should include lean protein, like fish, meat and eggs, low fat dairy, balanced with a variety of vegetables, salad and carbohydrates for good health and only a small amount of fats and sugars.

Aim to include each day:

- Two to three portions of protein, including fish, casseroled meat, pureed beans and pulses, eggs, and low fat cheese, milk and yoghurt.
- Three to five portions of vegetables and fruit for vitamins and fibre. This can include one small cup of dilute fruit juice each day.
- Two to three servings of low fat dairy for calcium, protein and minerals.
- Starchy carbohydrates including potato, bread, pasta, rice and cereal for energy, fibre, vitamins and minerals. They are low in fat unless you add butter, margarine or oil. Some people find it difficult to tolerate bread, pasta and rice after surgery; these need to be cooked well and chewed carefully to avoid discomfort.

- You need a little fat in your diet for vitamin A, D and E, but restrict butter, margarine and oils to three to four teaspoons a day. Avoid cream, processed foods, crisps and savoury pastries which all contain high levels of fat.
- Keep down your consumption of sugar and sweet foods, which are high in calories and contain few nutrients. You *cannot* rely on the surgery to do this for you so be vigilant of the amount of sugary foods you're including in your diet. Gastric bypass patients may experience an unpleasant reaction to sugary foods, known as dumping syndrome.

Keep up your fluid intake to prevent dehydration and constipation. Be guided by your thirst, but don't wait too long between drinks. Have around three pints of water, low sugar squash or tea and coffee, plus some semi-skimmed milk a day.

> [The hardest thing is] not being able to have a drink with my meal . . . I enjoy a glass of fruit juice with my meal and I miss it. I also miss not being able to gulp a drink and feel like my thirst is quenched immediately . . . [I need] lots of little sips to feel satisfied.
>
> K, gastric bypass

Frequent vomiting is not considered an inevitable part of life after weight loss surgery and can lead to problems such as band slippage, nutritional problems, damage to the oesophagus and tooth decay. Vomiting is usually due to eating or drinking too quickly or too much, or choosing textured foods, that cannot be easily chewed down, too soon after surgery.

Adjusting to your new relationship with food

In the weeks and months after surgery you will be adjusting to a very different way of approaching food. The restriction on food intake created by surgery will give you strong feedback on what and how much you can eat. Feelings of hunger are weakened and satiety signals are clearer; you should feel full on much smaller amounts of food and less hungry between meals. If you eat too much, or the wrong kinds of food, you may experience vomiting, abdominal pain or discomfort, bloating or dumping syndrome (the experience of nausea, faintness and diarrhoea that occurs in gastric bypass patients if they have sugary foods).

> I ate a tiny bit of chicken and chewed well. The pain was intense and I completely obstructed . . . I vomited but could not remove the

obstruction. I nearly had to go to hospital as the pain was 9/10 . . .
I am not now looking forward to eating solid food

N, gastric bypass

Many patients find that staple foods like bread, rice, pasta and meat, are difficult to tolerate and so need to experiment to find a range of foods that work for them and which provide a healthy, balanced diet. A degree of trial and error in what works for you is normal, but you need to avoid repeatedly 'testing the boundaries' of the surgical restriction.

Now I'm not on pure liquids . . . I'm not sure on what portions sizes to dish out to myself.

A, gastric band

How you respond to this new relationship with food will be a major factor in how successful you are with surgery. Some patients who struggle with the transition back to solid foods rely too heavily on soft foods and puddings that may be high in sugar and fat. Others may simply accept repeated vomiting rather than giving up the foods they enjoy. Both these scenarios are associated with poor weight loss and higher risk of complications.

The food I like now is completely different to the food I liked before
. . . I didn't have a sweet tooth before [but now] I do tend to eat
sweeter things because they are easier to digest . . . savoury things
like meat, cheese rolls, bacon rolls, proper dinners like steak and
kidney pie and vegetables I find them difficult to eat . . .I loved
salads before . . .I can't eat a salad now.
Gastric band patient quoted in Ogden *et al.* 2006: 284[2]

As well as the physical effect of restricted food intake, you will also need to adjust to the emotional impact of the loss of food for comfort and pleasure.

I felt bereft. That enjoyment from shopping, from the rituals of
buying, cooking and eating food were gone. It was a horrible feeling.
Food was my crutch and it had been taken away.
Lizzie Lee, gastric bypass patient, quoted in
Times Magazine, p29[4]

The psychological consequences of suddenly having food removed as a source of comfort may be particularly pronounced if you have a history of emotional eating.

Before [food] was this wonderful thing that tasted nice and made me feel good; very much a comforting and joyous thing and now it's just a pain in the arse, it really is. And it doesn't give me the satisfaction that it used to.

Gastric bypass patient quoted in
Ogden et al. 2011: 958[5]

Your new approach to eating will set the tone of your future relationship with food. This relationship may be positive, allowing you to lose a good amount of weight, feeling released from the tyranny of food and able instead to eat in response to hunger and nutritional need. Or it may be less helpful, as old patterns of eating re-emerge threatening the outcome of surgery. Bariatric dietitians sometimes talk of patients being 'too reliant on the surgical restriction', when patients assume that the restriction will always do the work for them. In reality the powerful feedback you get after surgery, the messages that prevent you from eating too much, diminish in the longer term and once again you will need to actively manage your food choices. Ultimately the question you face is – if I only have capacity for very little food what will I use food for, will it be for health, for pleasure or comfort? [2]

[Over the years] I have learnt a huge amount about my [eating] behaviours . . .I don't now rely 100% on the band as a crutch. Perhaps in the past two years I have valued it more as the tool it is. I have changed but I am not cured. This is a life-long journey emotionally [and] physically.

Gastric band patient and bariatric professional

General principles for eating after weight loss surgery

Weight loss surgery won't suddenly turn you into a restrained eater who only ever wants healthy foods. When people don't achieve good weight loss after surgery they often attribute this to a 'failure' of surgery to provide sufficient restriction; they expect the surgery to entirely control their eating and do not see themselves as having personal responsibility for how they use the 'tool' of surgery.[5]

I wouldn't even expect the bypass operation to be the be all and end of it. You've still got to use it as a tool to aid in your fight against weight. So I'm always going to have that problem of weight, always, always. And if I'm not careful, I could potentially go back to where I was.

Gastric band patient who underwent revision to
sleeve gastrectomy, quoted in Ogden et al. 2011: 959[5]

The benefits of exercise

> After the first 2 days at home, I was walking short distances to
> build my strength up and to get some exercise.
>
> K, gastric bypass

A number of studies, mainly looking at gastric bypass patients,
have a found an association between exercise levels and weight loss[9]
12 months after surgery. One meta-analysis (where researchers combine the results of lots of studies to see if they still get a helpful result)
suggests that people who keep up a reasonable level of physical exercise after surgery lose on average 4 per cent more BMI points than
non-exercisers.[10] Minimal exercise on the other hand is linked to poor
weight loss (less than 20 per cent excess weight) and gastric band
removal.[11,12] Of course, it may be that the people who lose more weight
after surgery feel better able to exercise or indeed that the people who
are exercising are generally more motivated so are better at sticking to
the correct diet, so we can't know for sure that it's exercise that offers
the extra weight loss, but it makes sense that maintaining good levels
of physical activity promotes weight loss as well as offering greater
physical and emotional well-being. Exercising regularly at a reasonable intensity boosts motivation and improves quality of life[13] and
reduces stress and depression.[14,15]

Most bariatric patients report an increase in physical activity post-
surgery, but people tend to be overgenerous when estimating time
spent exercising and find it hard to judge how much physical activity is
enough.[16] Below are some general ideas to help you think about
increasing physical activity, but you may need to speak to your GP to
check what exercise is suitable.

Exercise recommendations

There are three important components of a more active life: (i) reduced
sedentary time; (ii) a more active lifestyle; and (iii) regular exercise. All
three are required to promote weight loss, improve fitness and reduce
health problems after surgery. Try to set yourself a goal in each area,
one to decrease sitting time, one to encourage more activity in your
daily life and one related to exercise levels. You can build on these goals
as you lose weight and feel your fitness improving.

Reducing sedentary time

Physical activity is only one part of what's needed to get fitter and
reduce health risks. You also need to think about cutting down on
sedentary time. Sedentary time – meaning time spent sitting or lying

down, including sitting at a desk, working on a computer, driving, watching television or reading – is bad for your health and uses up very few calories. High levels of sedentary behaviour are a risk factor for coronary heart disease and diabetes[17] and each hour of daily television viewing is associated with an 11 per cent increase in mortality regardless of activity levels.[18]

To reduce sedentary time, you can:

- Break up sitting time with tasks that involve moving around.
- Walk to a colleague's desk rather than sending an email at work.
- Use ad breaks as a cue to get up, stretch and walk around the room.
- Set yourself daily limits on screen time – watching television or using the computer.
- Stand up or walk around the room when talking on the phone.
- Use a timer on the computer or your phone at work to remind you to stand up regularly.
- Walk short journeys rather than driving.

Increasing lifestyle activity

Increasing lifestyle activity is about incorporating physical activity in small, manageable blocks within your daily routine, so you are exercising without thinking about it. Look for ways to add in physical activity through your day so you accumulate active minutes; you won't need to worry so much about setting aside time for exercise as you're getting your activity levels up naturally through the day.

Think about the following:[19]

- Getting off the bus a couple of stops early.
- Using the stairs instead of the lift or stop the lift one floor below and walk up one flight of stairs.
- At the supermarket, park your car some distance from the entrance.
- Go for a walk during your lunch break.
- Do a little gardening regularly – your neighbours will be impressed and you'll get some exercise.
- Arrange to see your friends for a walk in the park rather than in a cafe for a coffee.

Exercise

The amount of physical exercise you can manage will depend on your existing fitness levels and health problems, gradually building up your fitness to improve health and well-being. In the long term you want to aim for the recommended level of exercise for adults[8] which is 150 minutes of moderate to vigorous physical activity accumulated over the week in bouts of ten minutes or more. Ideally this should include exercises that help strengthen muscle and bone, such as walking, climbing stairs, skipping or resistance training, a couple of days each week. Older people also benefit from exercises that improve balance, such as Tai Chi, to help prevent falls. The 150 active minutes can be achieved through formal exercise, such as exercise classes, swimming or sports, or through lifestyle activities such as gardening, walking the dog or dancing, but should be over and above your normal physical activity of everyday life, like walking around the shops.

If you have been relatively inactive before surgery, you will first of all need to focus on establishing physical activity as a life habit, setting realistic goals and gradually increasing the duration, frequency and intensity of exercise as you improve in fitness. Have you struggled to maintain regular exercise in the past? Spend some time thinking about why that was; what were the blocks that made exercise difficult? Was it that you felt self-conscious? That you got hot, uncomfortable and out of breath (which is pretty normal when you exercise vigorously, but you may need to build up your fitness first)? Are you worried about your health and whether it's safe to exercise? Is it difficult for you to get to a park or gym? Do you find it hard to make time between work and family commitments? These are real hurdles, but there may be ways around them. When you decided to have surgery, you made a commitment (to yourself, your family and your bariatric team) to do everything you could to make it successful and that includes physical activity on a regular basis. So when you've identified the main blocks, use a problem-solving technique to find a way to overcome them.

Problem solving involves writing down all the solutions you can think of and rating each potential solution on the basis of how helpful it is and on how difficult it would be to carry out. Of course some solutions are reasonably straightforward; for example if you're worried that your heart problem or arthritis will be made worse through exercise, then you need to talk to your GP. Others, such as difficulty accessing a park, gym or swimming pool because of where you live, may require more creative solutions.

So, for example, if the problem is that you find it hard to make time for exercise because you're with the children or working long hours, you could think about:

- Asking your partner or friend to look after the children a few times each week.
- Taking the whole family for a bike ride or to play tennis or football in the park.
- Asking your employer to let you have flexible hours so you can swim before work.

- Finding a gym with a crèche.
- Walking or cycling to work.

Try to think up as many solutions as possible and only when you've got a good list start to whittle it down to one or two of the best options. Decide on your preferred strategy, one that's realistic, and monitor the outcome. If it works, that's great, but if not, go back to your original list and try the next most helpful, realistic solution.

The most important aspect of exercise is that it's *regular* and *realistic*. There's little point in setting yourself a goal of going to the gym for an hour five times a week if you can't keep it up for more than a couple of weeks. If you set yourself up for failure it will leave you demoralised and less able to make the changes you need. Remember that even small changes in your activity levels can make an important difference.

Walking is one of the safest and easiest ways of establishing a realistic exercise habit. The general guidelines are that you should aim for 70,000–100,000 steps a week. This level of activity has been shown to enable people to lose between 2–8 per cent of their body weight *even without surgery*[20] so would definitely be a good start to promoting weight loss and improving fitness after surgery. Walking has the benefits of not requiring any special equipment (other than a comfortable pair of shoes and possibly a pedometer – see Chapter 5) and doesn't cost anything.

When planning exercise, think about the following:

- Find activities that you enjoy; group classes, swimming, aquaerobics, dancing and cycling are all excellent exercise.
- Create a habit of being more active rather than starting with an overambitious fitness plan.
- Set realistic short-term goals; having success with reasonable goals helps keep you motivated. If you set goals that are too difficult you'll set yourself up for failure and make it harder to stay focussed and motivated.
- Set time goals, not speed or distance goals. It's the time spent exercising that has the most impact on your health and you can increase the exercise intensity as you feel able.
- Monitor the intensity of exercise. Moderate to vigorous exercise should cause you to become a little out of breath, but you should still be able to have a conversation (known as the *talk test*). As you become fitter you will be able to do more intense exercise without getting too out of breath.
- Encourage family or friends to exercise with you.

If you are really struggling to motivate yourself to exercise, use this simple strategy to get yourself back on track. Agree with yourself a simple undemanding task, a five-minute walk or a ten-minute swim, that you feel confident about managing. This gets you back into exercise without the sense of it being a major burden, so allowing you a way to ease back into healthy habits. Also once you've started you may well find that it's not so bad after all and end up doing more. You may want to give yourself *credits* every time you meet your exercise goal and use these credits to earn yourself a treat, such as a new pair of shoes or a trip to the cinema.

Goal-setting and monitoring

Setting clear and realistic goals and keeping a record of your progress is one of the most effective ways of establishing a new, more active lifestyle. As with keeping a food diary (see Chapter 5), the process of recording and monitoring changes can be a very powerful tool. From a psychological point of view, writing things down makes them real and manageable; your exercise diary allows you to see the progress you've made and encourages the development of a healthy habit. Keep your diary somewhere convenient and obvious, by the front door or even next to the TV. If you're keen on technology, there are various exercise apps available for your smart phone.

Table 8.1 is an example of an exercise diary, setting out goals relating to reducing sedentary time, increasing lifestyle activity and more formal exercise, being clear about how often you plan to carry out the activity over the week. This example is for someone who is already pretty active and it may be that your own activity plan is less intense, particularly if you have health problems or a disability. Remember that any increase in physical activity is of benefit and it's important to start at the level that's right for you.

At the end of each week, review your activity diary. How did you get on; were the goals realistic or had you set them too high? If necessary adjust your goals so that you feel very confident that they're manageable. You also need to accept that there will always be times when life commitments get in the way of exercise goals. Just make a note of what got in the way; if it happens a lot and threatens to derail your plan use the problem-solving technique to find a way around the problem. It may be that you need to re-think when or how you do exercise.

How can I increase my chances of success?

Changing unhelpful habits

As we have seen in this chapter there are a whole set of adjustments that you need to make to your eating habits and lifestyle to be success-ful with weight loss surgery. These changes may involve breaking

Table 8.1 An exercise diary

Date	Anti-sedentary goal	Active lifestyle goal		Exercise goal
	Television – less than 1½ hours Aim: daily	20 minute walk during lunch break Aim: 4–5 days/wk	Walk up and down stairs at home/work Aim: 5 × day	Swimming 30 minutes Aim: 2 × week
Mon	✓	✓	✓	
Tues	✓	✓	✓	
Wed	✓		✓	✓
Thurs	✓	✓	✓	
Fri	✓	✓	✓	
Sat			✓	✓
Sun	✓		✓	✓
Notes	Tired after going swimming on Saturday and wanted to relax with the family. Still did really well.	Only missed Wednesday because of a work meeting, but was able to go swimming with the kids after work instead.	No problem – will aim for 6 times next week.	Even better than planned because I went swimming on Wednesday. Twice a week is realistic though.

long-standing habits or making profound changes to the way you think about day-to-day activities and choices. In this next section we will look at the skills you may need to make these important changes.

The patients who are successful for many years after gastric bypass are those who are able to maintain a set of helpful habits. If success is defined as keeping off three-quarters of initial weight loss, successful patients all tend to demonstrate the same pattern of behaviours; eating three meals a day with just one or two snacks, avoiding fizzy drinks and alcohol, getting plenty of sleep, taking vitamin and mineral supplements, exercising a number of times each week and having a strong sense of their personal responsibility for maintaining their weight.[21]

Perhaps unsurprisingly, many people struggle to make these changes to long-standing habits of eating. Some studies suggest that over a third of weight loss surgery patients are unable or unwilling to comply with the changes to diet and lifestyle changes recommended by their bariatric team, usually by snacking, having too large portions, failure to increase physical activity, not taking nutritional supplements, or consuming too much alcohol.[22, 23] The result of this is poor weight loss or weight regain; ten years after surgery 25 per cent of gastric band and almost 10 per cent of gastric bypass patients are back to within 5 per cent of their original, pre-surgery weight.[24]

People are creatures of habit and habits are hard to change. But what is a habit? Simply put, a habit is a behaviour performed repeatedly in the same environment or location. Habits develop naturally over time as people go about their everyday lives. By their nature habits are quick to activate – that is the habitual behaviour will win over alternative behaviours – and people value these repetitive behaviours because they feel familiar and easy. In this way habits offer *the path of least resistance* as we go about our lives. Habits are also slow to extinguish; the memory trace of the habitual behaviour hangs around for a long time, which is why breaking a habit can feel like a long and arduous task. Lack of time, distraction and lowered self-control (due to other demands or stresses) all increase the likelihood of acting on a habit.[25]

One example of a habit, studied by psychologists in California, was eating popcorn at the cinema.[25] In this scenario the habitual behaviour could be described as 'I eat popcorn when I go to the cinema'. In this study some of the fresh, tasty popcorn was replaced with week-old, stale popcorn. What the researchers discovered was that the habitual popcorn eaters ate as much stale popcorn as fresh popcorn, even though they found it less appetising. Non-habitual popcorn eaters disliked the stale popcorn and so consumed less of it.

If you like to snack on your favourite crisps while watching television or you always have a cake and coffee at the cafe when you meet your friend on a Wednesday morning, you have food habits that could cause problems after surgery. The same applies to physical activity habits; if you always come home from a hard day at work looking forward to a cup of tea and a sit down, it will be hard to establish a new routine of stopping off at the gym or going for a walk around the block. The reality is that most of us have unhelpful food or lifestyle habits that feel comfortable and easy. Breaking out of these habits after surgery is likely to be one of your major challenges.

Changing old habits and developing new habits requires repeated experience of the new behaviour to develop new habit memories. People are helped to break habits by carefully monitoring their behaviour to prevent slips; by having an intention to behave differently; and by changing the environment so the habit is less likely to be activated.

Self-monitoring

One of the best strategies for breaking unhelpful habits is vigilant monitoring.[26] By keeping careful focus on the behaviour, we increase self-control and inhibit the mindless activation of habitual behaviour. Keeping a detailed food dairy (as described in Chapter 5) is a way of distancing yourself from your own behaviour. By recording the amount and type of food you eat, as well as information about the time, place and feelings, you are able to become aware of previously unrecognised eating behaviour. Knowing that you have to write it down in your food diary will make you more conscious of what you're eating and may help strengthen your resolve to stick to a healthier diet.

The rules about self-monitoring apply to other behaviours; if you want to reduce the amount of time spent watching television or playing computer games; start walking every day or get to an exercise class; drink less alcohol; be more sociable; eat more fruit; or take your children swimming, all these behaviours can be monitored and recorded, giving you a better chance of developing a successful new habit.

Reinforce your good intentions

Implementation intentions are a conscious decision to behave in a different way in a particular situation. They work best when paired with high levels of personal motivation and when you also make changes to your environment. Their main value is in reminding you what you've decided to do (your intention) so making you less liable to fall back on your habitual behaviour.

You need to have a clear idea of what you want to do and plan the exact situation where you are going to perform the behaviour. It's important to visualise the scene where you will be carrying out the new behaviour, whether in the gym, a restaurant or supermarket.[27] Support your goal by having a clearly defined intention, such as: 'If it's Thursday morning I'll go for a run for half an hour.'

The behavioural intention is particularly important if you're feeling angry or upset.[28] People are more likely to make risky decisions if they are in a bad mood; the 'to hell with it' effect can lead you to make poor choices. You can minimise the effect of mood on behaviour by having a plan already in place. It's been suggested that the average person makes over 250 decisions about food each day:[29] Shall I skip breakfast? Should I take food into work with me? Should I have crumble or yoghurt for pudding? Decide in advance what you will do in each scenario, such as: 'Every workday I'll get up 30 minutes earlier to have breakfast' or 'When I go to the canteen I will choose my lunch from the salad bar'. Remember to picture yourself doing the action to increase the strength of the intention.

Change the environment

While self-control, monitoring and good intentions can get us so far, we are vulnerable to fluctuations in willpower.[30] While you can't rely on self-control for permanent behaviour change, it can offer a window of opportunity for other longer-term strategies[25] in particular changes to the environment.

Use your food diary to think about the *environment cues* that impact on your eating. Do you snack in front of the television? Do you grab a bag of crisps or a chocolate bar while waiting to pay at the petrol station? These environment cues are situations or places that trigger a habitual eating behaviour. You can start to break a habit by making changes to your environment so the habit memory is less likely to be activated.

The following are the kinds of changes that may help:

- Move your furniture so your regular 'snacking chair' is in a different place.
- Change the way you shop. When we go to a supermarket we all tend to walk up the same aisles and reach for the same kinds of food; help yourself make different food choices by going to a different, unfamiliar supermarket where you will be less driven by habitual responses.
- Change the way you carry out the behaviour. In the cinema study described above, habitual popcorn eaters ate less stale popcorn if they were instructed to eat with their left hand. By eating with a different hand it made them more conscious of, and able to modify, their behaviour. So if you took the example of altering your shopping habits, perhaps rather than change supermarket, you could simply start shopping from the other end of the store.
- Only take enough money out with you each day to cover your necessary expenses. Don't carry cards that allow you to shop freely.
- Avoid social situations where you are liable to overeat. For example, buffet restaurants encourage people to eat more than they want or need, if only to 'get their money's worth'.
- It's important to remove temptation from the environment, so don't keep snack food in the house; having access to large amounts of snack foods simply increases the likelihood of overeating.
- Limit the time and place of eating. It's helpful to have an agreement in the family that you only eat at the table to reduce thoughtless snacking and break the association between food and other activities.

Reward yourself for work well done

Build in a reward for your achievements, whether it's increased exercise, changed eating habits, giving up smoking, reducing your consumption of alcohol or practising relaxation or stress management skills. Make sure the reward is for a change of behaviour rather than weight loss itself – it's the new behaviours that will give you the best outcome in the long term when the surgical weight loss has slowed. You can reward yourself using tokens that build up to earn a treat or social rewards (in the same way teachers use gold stars to reward hard-working and well behaved children). You can be as creative as you want in devising your reward system, but avoid using food rewards for obvious reasons.

Accept support from other people

Social support is important for everyone and even more so if we are facing major life challenges. Encouragement and support from family and friends helps to maintain motivation and commitment. Attending a bariatric support group has also been shown to be helpful and the advice and understanding from people who are in the same boat may help you achieve better weight loss.[31, 32] Where people do not feel they are getting sufficient support from their family or bariatric team, support groups become even more important.

> I am getting 'reflux' which burns my throat and have not even bothered to phone the [private] surgeon's office after the last reply I got. But at the meeting I was advised to take a particular drug that helps with the burning . . . thank God for the support group.
>
> J, sleeve gastrectomy

After a year or so, family and friends are likely to be less demonstrative in their backing.[33] From their perspective you've been through the difficult bit, you've made the changes and lost the weight so your need for ongoing support may not be so evident. Use the assertiveness skills you learnt in Chapter 6 to be clear with family and friends about your needs and wants.

> [and] people also quickly forget so now I still get served far too much food or family and friends regularly forget the foods I can't eat very well or how things need to be cooked.
>
> A, gastric bypass

Avoid being hampered by embarrassment or politeness from stating what you do or don't need and keep your requests clear and straightforward, for example:[34]

- Do not eat snack food in front of me.
- Do not bring unhealthy food into the house.
- Respect my efforts to change the way I eat.
- Don't tempt me with unhealthy foods.
- Remind me of my goals and distract me if I weaken.

Challenge unhelpful thinking

Becoming more aware of unhelpful patterns of thinking about your relationship with food can help you maintain a more helpful perspective on a situation or problem. By challenging self-defeating thoughts you can feel more able to cope with difficulties you face after surgery. When you feel tempted to give up on a diet or activity goal, try to identify the underlying thought that is getting in the way of positive change and the feeling attached to the thought, be it sadness, anxiety, frustration or anger. Ask yourself, is this thinking helpful for me? Would I think like this if I wasn't upset? Are there other possible explanations for the situation other than the one that is making me feel sad, fearful or angry? Am I thinking about the world as if there are rules about how things *should* be? Am I under-estimating my ability to cope with this? Use these questions to create a more helpful, alternative thought. As with all these new skills it works best if you regularly write down your thoughts in a diary.

Often people with a long history of dieting have a number of unhelpful thinking habits. Steinberg and Dryden (1996)[34] offer examples of common self-defeating thoughts experienced by people trying to manage their eating and the *positive self-talk* they can use to challenge this thinking (Table 8.2).

Do these thoughts sound familiar to you? If you identify a powerful self-defeating thought that often becomes fixed in your mind, write down the more helpful response and keep it with you. Try also to identify any unhelpful thoughts about exercising, like 'I can barely walk to the end of the road, I'll never be able to get fitter' or 'Gyms are only for beautiful people who have never had to manage their weight', and challenge these as well.

Keep in mind your reasons for choosing weight loss surgery

Patients often tell me that, of course, they'll stick to all the rules after surgery; why would you put yourself though the risk and discomfort of surgery just to blow it all eating the wrong foods again? But it's always easier to feel determined before the event; think about times when you've gone to a restaurant resolute about not ordering the chocolate cake or your best intentions to go to the gym tomorrow morning. As we have seen earlier in this chapter, faced with day-to-day reality human beings struggle to maintain their motivation and the pull of old habits can be immense. Do not deceive yourself that it will be fine because you are so grateful for being given weight loss surgery or because you will feel so great once you start losing weight. The motivational value of gratitude and the buzz of weight loss can readily become lost in daily life as you try to balance the challenges of surgery against the normal demands and difficulties of everyday existence.

Table 8.2 Challenging self-defeating thoughts

Self-defeating thought	Alternative, helpful response
'I can't stand being deprived.'	'I don't like being deprived, but I can stand it. I'm able to cope with more than I think.'
'Why do I have to be the only one having to watch what I eat? I hate being different.'	'I don't like being different and limited in my food choices, but really it's not that terrible. I need to remember my goals.'
'This should be easier, not such a constant effort.'	'Why should something that's hard be easier just because I ask it to be? It's hard because it's hard, but I decided to make a go of it and I will succeed if I persevere.'
'I'm so anxious, I need to eat – it's the only way to feel better.'	'Eating won't get rid of my anxiety; it will just distract me for a short time and will give me additional problems to handle. I can tolerate some anxiety and find a better way to deal with it.'
'It's impossible, I'll never succeed!'	'This may be very difficult at times, but difficult doesn't mean impossible. I need to remember my strengths and focus on my goals.'
'I had some cake at the office party, I'm a failure. I don't deserve to succeed!'	'Just because I had a slip doesn't mean I'm a failure as a person and I've had many successes in my life. A failure in the past doesn't stop me succeeding in the future.'
'I want that food. I must have it now.'	'I don't need everything that I simply want. It's hard to pass up lovely food, but I'll feel better if I do.'
'I can't stand this frustration.'	'I can stand a little frustration, even though it's unpleasant. It's a part of life and I can still enjoy myself in many ways.'

As you lose weight it's easy to forget how you felt before surgery – the self-consciousness, feeling out of breath walking down the street, the anxiety about your health, facing negative comments from other people – and start to take the improvements in your health and quality of life for granted. And from taking it from granted, it's a short step to becoming dissatisfied; that you are not as slim as you wanted to be or that your life isn't as great after surgery as you had imagined. This dissatisfaction can cause you to become demoralised, losing sight of great changes you have achieved and vulnerable to a return to problematic eating. So what can you do?

You can also try writing a list of all the ways your weight affects you now, before surgery, in as much detail as possible and including the emotional impact of these difficulties or limitations (Table 8.3). It may feel painful but it will give you a snapshot of the impact of the weight on your life now. You'll be able to return to this list in the future, if you're feeling disappointed with your progress, and acknowledge just how far you've come.

Table 8.3 Impact of weight

How my weight affects me now

Georgina S   Date March 2011

Problem	Impact on my life . . .	Impact on how I feel . . .
Not being able to get into airplane seats etc	Miss out on holidays with family. I definitely can't take the children to Thorpe Park.	Sad and frustrated. Feel like I'm not able to do things that normal people do.
Diabetes	Have to take medication all the time and test my blood sugars.	Was very upset when diagnosed with diabetes. It was proof that my weight was out of control. My doctor told me about the risks of having diabetes and now feel very VERY anxious about my health.
Get short of breath and hot and uncomfortable if I do anything active.	I can't do things with the children that I'd like – playing in the park. Even the weekly shop is difficult. Not able to manage any exercise that could help me manage my weight.	Feel trapped in my body. It won't do what I want it to do and there doesn't seem any possibility of being able to get fitter. It's embarrassing to even walk around the block because I'm huffing and puffing.
Not being able to shop on the high street.	Have to buy expensive clothes from plus size shops online or just make do with what I already have – nothing looks good on me anyway. I have wardrobes full of clothes that don't fit me.	I feel ugly and ashamed, like I don't deserve nice clothes.
Hate my appearance and can't look in a mirror.	Spend my life trying to cover up my body. Can't do anything, like swimming, that involves getting undressed. Try to avoid seeing my reflection if I'm out and horrified if I catch a glimpse of myself.	Sometimes feel completely disgusted with my body. I hate the way I look and can't see why my husband could ever find me attractive.
The whole problem with food.	I feel preoccupied with food and my next meal. I feel hungry all the time.	I hate being controlled by food – it's like it doesn't matter if I'm happy or sad, I always want to eat. And when I eat I feel disgusted that I can't stop.

Some people also find it useful to keep a journal of their journey through weight loss surgery; it provides a record of the changes in your life and supports your ongoing commitment. A number of websites allow you to track your weight post-surgery, but beware of fixating on weight loss rather than improvements in health and quality of life. Sooner or later the weight loss will stop and if that's the only thing keeping you motivated you might run into problems. Basing progress on your physical and emotional well-being, your ability to get out in the world and do the things you want to do, will provide a more lasting motivation.

Summary

- Making a success of weight loss surgery is major challenge, requiring you to make life-long changes to the way you eat and your lifestyle choices. While it can offer great benefits to health, quality of life and emotional well-being, these come at a cost of a lot of hard work. The patients that do best are those who take responsibility for making these changes happen, rather than relying on the *magic* of surgery.
- In the weeks following surgery you will need to follow a liquid diet, only slowly moving onto soft food and then a more regular healthy diet. This process allows the body time to heal and moving too quickly on to solid foods will increase the risk of complications.
- Being more active promotes quicker weight loss and improved physical and emotional well-being. It's helpful to set goals to reduce sedentary time, increase lifestyle activity and incorporate regular exercise into your weekly schedule.
- Habits offer *the path of least resistance* and long-established habits can be hard to break. You can support your new habits by keeping a food and physical activity diary; being very clear about your intentions; and by making changes to the environment. Reward yourself for healthy behaviours.
- Access help and encouragement by joining a support group. Be clear with friends and family about how they can best support you by making direct, assertive requests.
- Identify and challenge unhelpful thoughts that create frustration and upset and block positive change.
- Before surgery write down the ways in which your health, lifestyle and emotional well-being are affected by your weight and keep a record of your weight loss journey to bolster your commitment to change.

Stories in the media and online often present a polarised view of weight loss surgery. On the one hand they champion surgery as a magical gateway to a new life, offering up a picture of people who lose all their excess weight, start a new happy relationship, are offered the job of their dreams and run a marathon. On the other hand, horror stories tell of people left unable to eat anything or still all too able to eat, of people whose relationships break down or who sell their house to fund cosmetic surgery. The reality for most weight loss surgery patients, of course, falls somewhere between these two extremes. Most patients achieve reasonable weight loss, have better health and greater confidence, but this is balanced by the stress of coping with unpleasant symptoms and the challenge of making radical changes in their relationship with food. Over the next two chapters we will look more closely at these positive outcomes and also the more difficult problems or complications that patients sometimes face.

9

'It's the best decision I ever made': success stories with weight loss surgery

'I now feel positive that I can succeed . . .'

N, gastric bypass

There is a lot of variation in people's responses to surgery and this is reflected in outcome – both in weight loss and patient satisfaction. While some people do exceptionally well, lose a great deal of weight and feel better physically and emotionally, there are also patients who don't do so well. So, which patients tend to do best? If you ask bariatric teams who they like to see in clinic, they are pretty clear about which patients are most successful.

The patient all bariatric teams like to see is the one who has made up her own mind (we'll assume it's a woman for now, but it's equally true for men) about having weight loss surgery. She is looking to surgery to improve her health and quality of life, rather than primarily to improve her appearance. She arrives motivated and well informed, having a clear understanding of the process and good insight into the potential challenges and difficulties. She will have done her research and may have spoken to other weight loss surgery patients. She understands that the surgery is not magic, has realistic weight loss expectations and knows that she will need to make life-long changes to eating habits. Importantly she sees the process of weight loss surgery as a *partnership* between herself and the bariatric team – both sharing responsibility for ensuring the best outcome.

The successful patient is likely to have good support from family and friends. She will be open and honest about her eating habits and is able to make changes to her eating in preparation for surgery. After surgery, the main factors that influence her success will be her ability (and willingness) to stick to the dietary recommendations, her persistence with a routine of physical activity, regular monitoring of food intake and exercise, and conscientiousness when it comes to attending follow-up appointments with the bariatric team.[1]

What are the benefits of weight loss surgery?

There is no doubt that people who do well with weight loss surgery report high levels of satisfaction. Weight loss surgery can enable you to lose between 20 per cent (gastric band) and 30 per cent (with gastric bypass) of your initial weight. Weight stabilises after a number of years and, even with some weight regain, at ten years post-surgery patients can remain 14–25 per cent below their original, pre-surgery weight.[2] This degree of weight loss is far greater than most people can expect to maintain after a conventional weight management programme and can produce dramatic improvements in health, life expectancy, social functioning and emotional well-being.

Improvements in health and life expectancy

While we still need rigorous, long-term evidence from randomised controlled trials (the best kind of research for showing the effectiveness of treatment) on the health and quality of life benefits[3], all the evidence so far suggests that the level of weight loss produced by bariatric surgery results in excellent improvements in a range of health problems associated with obesity.

Generally speaking, improvements in comorbidities are determined by the extent of weight loss achieved, with better weight loss producing greater health benefits. Even a loss of 10 per cent body weight produces meaningful improvements in cardiovascular risk, diabetes, hypertension and dyslipidaemia.[4]

> The first 3st came off fairly quickly and I felt the benefit of that . . . and that kept me going. The heart palpitations, sleep apnoea, the pain in the feet and ankles ALL GONE after 5st.
>
> J, sleeve gastrectomy

Diabetes. All bariatric procedures can result in good improvement in type 2 diabetes and insulin resistance; across all procedures 75 per cent of patients experience a complete resolution and more experience improvement of diabetes. Around 85 per cent of patients experience significant improvement or complete resolution of type 2 diabetes after gastric bypass,[5,6,7] 98 per cent with biliopancreatic diversion/duodenal switch,[8] 55–66 per cent with sleeve gastrectomy[7,9] and 44 per cent with the gastric band.[7] Remission of diabetes occurs faster with the malabsorptive procedures, gastric bypass and BPD/DS, than with the gastric band. While improved glycaemic control with gastric band is dependent on weight loss, with bypass and BPD/DS it occurs *before* significant weight loss, with almost half of all diabetic bypass patients showing improved insulin resistance within seven days of surgery due to changes in gastric neurohormones.[10] Gastric bypass is also more likely than the band to lead to complete remission, allowing you to come off all diabetic medication.

People who have had diabetes for longer may not see such good improvement compared with those who have a more recent diagnosis. Diabetes may also not resolve after surgery if you do not comply with the dietary guidelines or you have inadequate weight loss.[11]

Hypertension and dyslipidaemia. All bariatric procedures can produce improvements in the other components of metabolic syndrome – hypertension and dyslipidaemia. Around 60 per cent of all weight loss surgery patients show a complete resolution of hypertension with more showing improvement. For specific procedures, around 44 per cent of gastric band patients, 69 per cent of sleeve gastrectomy and 79 per cent of gastric bypass patients[7] show improvement or resolution of hypertension by one year after surgery.

Almost three-quarters of bariatric patients show lowered levels of 'bad' cholesterol and triglycerides and raised levels of 'good' cholesterol after surgery. As with diabetes and hypertension, the best results for normalisation of blood lipids is with BPD/DS and gastric bypass, followed by the sleeve gastrectomy and gastric band.[7]

Obstructive sleep apnoea. Over all procedures, two-thirds of sleep apnoea patients are able to come off treatment after bariatric surgery[5] again with improvements most pronounced in gastric bypass patients.

Other health problems. Weight loss surgery patients experience reduced bodily pain, including knee, ankle[12] and back pain.[13] Some 80 per cent of patients show improvement in non-alcoholic fatty liver disease[14] and 50–70 per cent reduced symptoms of reflux disease.[7,15]

Life expectancy

Because of its positive impact on various health risks, weight loss surgery is associated with greater life expectancy. Bariatric surgery reduces risk of death by all causes, and death due to cardiovascular disease,[16] compared with people who do not have surgery. Improvements in high blood pressure, type 2 diabetes, coronary heart disease, dyslipidaemia and sleep apnoea, and reduced risk of cancer, all contribute to a marked increase in life expectancy and it's been estimated that bariatric surgery reduces death *by any cause* by 40 per cent at seven years post-surgery.[17,18] Diabetic patients who go through weight loss surgery have 9 per cent mortality at nine years, compared with 28 per cent mortality for an equivalent non-surgical group of obese diabetics. Gastric bypass surgery has been shown to be associated with a

92 per cent decrease in death from diabetes, a 60 per cent reduction in death from cancer and 56 per cent reduction in death due to coronary artery disease,[17,18,19] though these benefits of reduced mortality may not be present for high risk older, male patients.[20]

Pregnancy and fertility[21]

Women are expected to avoid pregnancy during the period of rapid weight loss (up 18–24 months after surgery) as the body may not be getting sufficient nutrients to ensure that you and the baby are healthy. Weight loss after surgery is associated with a normalisation of hormonal balance and menstrual cycles and a reduction in polycystic ovary syndrome and so may have a positive effect on fertility. You may need to speak to your GP about contraception and take precautions against pregnancy even if you've previously been told that you can't get pregnant. If you do get pregnant you need to let you bariatric team know promptly so they can monitor you. There are studies showing successful pregnancies within one or two years of surgery, but there is a risk of nutritional deficiencies, particularly with gastric bypass and biliopancreatic diversion/duodenal switch (BPD/DS).

Most studies conclude that pregnancy after weight loss surgery is safe for both the mother and baby.[22] A number of studies have found lower rates of gestational diabetes, preeclampsia and pregnancy-induced hypertension in a bariatric group compared to a group of obese women who had not had surgery. However, among gastric bypass patients there is a risk of the baby having a neural tube defect if the mother fails to take the recommended vitamin supplements. Women who have had BPD/DS also need to be monitored very closely for nutritional deficiencies during pregnancy and there may be an increased risk of miscarriage in this group. Surgery does not appear to have a major effect on rates of caesarean section, with some studies showing it as more likely and some less likely following surgery.

Physical well-being

Along with resolution of comorbidities, for many patients there comes a great enhancement in physical well-being. As they lose weight patients often feel more energetic, they have less joint and back pain and are able to be active, so enabling a better quality of life.[23] One year after surgery almost 50 per cent of weight loss surgery patients report significant improvement in their ability to carry out day-to-day activities.[5] This rapid improvement in health and energy levels often in turn allows people to feel happier, offering a chance at a fresh start in life.

> I have more energy and can do more exercise. I feel happier in myself . . . more confident and enjoy it when people comment on

how well I am doing and how much weight I have lost now. I still have a long way to go, but I am happy.

K, gastric bypass

[I feel] . . . much happier, fitter and able to go and do.

J, sleeve gastrectomy

Improvements in emotional health, social functioning and quality of life

As well as better health and increased life expectancy, weight loss surgery can also enhance quality of life, general well-being, social confidence, emotional health and ability to take part in leisure activities.[24] People describe a normalisation of everyday activities, walking to the shop, having a bath, playing with your children or doing the housework,[25] that were effortful or stressful before surgery. Most studies find that bariatric patients report better quality of life, with sustained improvements in employment opportunities, relationships, anxiety and depression a number of years after surgery[26,27,28] with the degree of weight loss being the best predictor of enhanced quality of life.[29]

The changes in emotional well-being and fitness allow some patients to feel they can make a new start in life, perhaps one they had felt they would never achieve.

[I would like to have known] the long-term effects . . . even so I am not sure it would have stopped me if I had known, my life was almost not worth living before . . . it has given me my life back.

J, sleeve gastrectomy

I now feel positive that I can succeed. [Before] I felt that I would never achieve my goal due to all the numerous failures over the years.

N, gastric bypass

I feel much happier, although not 'all cured' yet.

J, gastric bypass

Escape from the tyranny of food

Food has no role in my life, it just has no meaning, I just don't think about it.

Gastric band patient quoted in Ogden *et al.* 2006: 285[30]

Many patients come to weight loss surgery feeling utterly powerless to manage their weight and seek to gain control through surgery. After bariatric surgery, patients often describe feeling less hungry, more in control of their eating and less vulnerable to binge episodes.[31] For this reason, surgery has been characterised as the finding of control through the removal of control;[30] by having the control over what and how they eat taken away, patients can paradoxically feel more in control of themselves and their lives, and most importantly in their relationship with food. They often experience reduced preoccupation with food and are freed from the constant nagging of hunger.

> Food no longer controls my life, I do not wake up thinking straightaway of food. I look at each meal as an important meal, and I eat slowly and stop as soon as I feel full. I don't ever overstuff as it feels uncomfortable and I feel very protective of my new stomach pouch that the surgeon gave me.
>
> K, gastric bypass

> I don't think about food all the time. Now I eat to live rather than the reverse.
>
> C, gastric bypass

> [Surgery] has given me a 'tool' to control my eating. I joined Weight Watchers in 1969; signed up with Dr . . . of Harley St in 1970 . . . signed up with . . . . in 1993 and went on to put on another 6 stones; [I] did the Cambridge, the cabbage soup diet, back to WeightWatchers, joined the gym, took up yoga, took up pilates . . . You name it NOTHING had the effect this operation has had.
>
> J, sleeve gastrectomy

Patients report less hunger, less disinhibition of eating and increased dietary restraint[32] and the diminished experience of hunger can feel hugely empowering for people who have experienced their lives dominated by a desire for food. Of course not all hunger is physical hunger, caused by having an empty stomach, but is often driven instead by seeking pleasure in the absence of physical need. Gastric bypass has been shown to decrease the experience of *hedonic hunger*,[33] the craving for highly palatable food often described by people with severe weight problems, probably due to changes in the neurohormones that control hunger and satiety.

> I have lost 2st 6lb in 6 weeks, I have found that I am not hungry and when I do eat I feel full quicker and for longer.
>
> K, gastric bypass

> [The best thing] is not feeling hungry anymore . . . I feel it gives me control over food which I didn't have before.
>
> N, gastric bypass

For some patients this imposed control comes with costs.

[Food is] not my 'friend' any more as it hurts if I overeat.

J, sleeve gastrectomy

Patients may remain aware of an issue in their emotional relationship with food. As a re-emergence of emotional or binge eating can lead to excessive weight regain months or years after surgery, it makes sense to try work to resolve these issues and develop other emotional management tools. Some researchers[34] believe that weight loss surgery patients who show binge eating should be offered psychological therapy after surgery to prevent it from derailing the surgical outcome.

I physically cannot eat [the food I used to eat] so I have to find other ways to cope with my life, which is why I am seeing an eating disorder counsellor . . .

J, gastric bypass

Ideally, bariatric patients move towards some degree of flexibility in the way they approach food, so their eating is not characterised by over-control or loss of control. This requires you to listen to your body, recognising and responding to feelings of hunger and satiety. However, not everyone finds that surgery gives them this sense of control. They may continue to feel hunger or struggle to manage emotional eating; this may emerge more strongly some time after surgery as the physical restriction on the amount eaten starts to lessen.

I have tried [to binge eat] but it is too painful so it has stopped me. Now I know how painful it is, it's not so satisfying to do . . . but I worry that the inclination is ever there . . . stress and working at home alone does not help, they seem to be the worst days.

J, sleeve gastrectomy

I still have bouts of sickness when I overeat

J, gastric bypass

I still eat bits of chocolate and crisps, just a taste. You just try to cheat it I suppose, it's part of the illness . . . [I am] more likely to eat the wrong things when upset or stressed or left alone.

J, gastric bypass

As they are so restricted in how much they can eat, patients are faced with a choice of what they will eat. Ultimately it will always be your choice as to whether you make the healthy choice or go for the tempting foods.

> I no longer crave sweet or fatty foods, because I know what that will do to me and I don't want this. I don't want to be obese anymore, I want to be healthy.
>
> K, gastric bypass

> I eat what I fancy but in small portions or as 'tastes'. I had this surgery to be NORMAL not to be confined and restricted for the rest of my life and feel guilty about looking at a certain food. I try to have a balance as has always been taught that one eats healthy and consistently throughout the day/week, but a treat . . . or something slightly different once in a while won't hurt. PLUS, I know from my own past that if I deprive myself of something for too long then I will binge on that item to the point of making myself sick.
>
> A, gastric bypass

Some people find that their tastes change completely, that they want to eat more healthily, are interested in the nutritional value of food, and hopefully begin to eat with more conscious awareness.

> My tastes are completely different . . . The major changes are I detest any fried foods like MacDonald's, fried chicken, bacon, I absolutely detest it . . . Everything I like is low calorie . . . All the fatty food I just don't like them.
>> Gastric bypass patient quoted in Ogden *et al*. 2006: 284[30]

> [the hardest part] was getting used to 'mindful eating'.
>
> C, gastric bypass

Emotional health

> My mood is a lot brighter, I don't worry that people will be looking at me when I am out or [that] they might shout fat comments at me, and if they do I feel emotionally strong enough to not care
>
> K, gastric bypass

Many weight loss surgery patients report that they feel less distressed and anxious and these improvements in emotional well-being can be sustained many years after surgery.[35] As with all the benefits from surgery, greater weight loss predicts more improvement in depression and anxiety.[36]

Studies have not been able to show a definite link between

depression before surgery and the success of surgery. At least one study[1] has found that higher depression scores pre-surgery are associated with *less* risk of significant weight regain. Other studies have suggested that people with high levels of depression and anxiety don't do as well as non-depressed patients. It has been suggested that where depression or other emotional problems are primarily due to the obesity (through the impact of obesity on self-esteem, quality of life and relationships for example) then it is likely to resolve following surgery. Where the emotional difficulties are unrelated to the weight issue and/or occurred before the weight problem they are less likely to improve spontaneously after surgery.[37] To this extent outcome would be determined by whether or not the person remains depressed after surgery or experiences an improvement in their mood and coping resources.

It may seem counterintuitive, but there are a number of possible reasons as to why low mood before surgery could be associated with a better outcome.[1] One explanation could be that weight loss leads quickly to improved mood, greater motivation and access to better emotional coping resources, allowing the patient to maintain healthy changes:

Helen had been feeling so low before surgery; her health problems meant she was unable to work and she felt lonely and purposeless. As she lost weight, she began to experience energy and motivation she hadn't felt for years. She started voluntary work at the local hospice and bloomed with a newfound sense of involvement and belonging. Her mood improved and, focusing on her goals, she was able to keep her meals managed and her eating controlled. Her busy schedule was very different from her sedentary lifestyle before surgery.

Alternatively, patients with depression pre-surgery may be more likely to get offered support in the way of psychological therapy or counselling and it is this that helps them sustain a healthier lifestyle over the months and years.

Frank had been depressed for years. Now 46, in his 30s he had gone through two redundancies, and felt low and hopeless about the future. His work and playing football had kept his weight in check when he was younger, but after he became depressed he stopped playing sport, avoided his friends and used food as a comfort. The medication they put him on seemed to make him feel hungry all the time, and besides there was nothing else to do. When he was seen by the bariatric team for assessment they were concerned that his long-standing depression would make it hard for him to cope after surgery and they suggested that he be referred for psychological therapy. In therapy, Bill started to recognise how he used food to suppress feelings of hurt and hopelessness. He developed new ways of coping with these feelings and slowly began to feel better. Avoiding comfort foods after surgery was a challenge, but he was helped by ongoing support from his therapist.

Or again, it could be that the most depressed people before surgery are also the ones who feel most determined to make a permanent change.

When she pictured her life, Sue imagined a plughole with her life rapidly disappearing down the hole. She was frightened when she thought of her increasing physical limitations, but despaired about her ability to make a difference. She came to weight loss surgery with her eyes open – she knew that it would be the hardest thing she had ever done, but she also felt strongly that it was her only chance. She applied herself to the task like a military campaign, planning every meal in advance; strictly controlling all foods that came in to the house; doing exercise every day and keeping a careful note of her achievements.

Helen, Frank and Sue all did well because they used surgery as a springboard from which to tackle big questions about what they wanted from life, how they saw themselves and how they dealt with difficult emotions, which in turn acted as a foundation for long-lasting changes in their relationship with food. However, if you continue to feel significantly depressed after surgery, it will sap your energy and motivation, make you less able to use the support of family and friends, and may increase emotional eating, making it difficult to maintain good weight loss. People who have a long history of major depression may continue to experience difficulties after surgery and it's important to seek help swiftly, initially from your GP. If you feel you would benefit from counselling or therapy there is information about how to access help in Chapter 11.

Self-esteem, body image and social confidence

Weight loss surgery patients speak of feeling more respected and valued by others,[30] with improved self-esteem, greater social confidence and an ability to be more assertive in their dealings with other people.[38] People often become more socially active, enjoying their new lease of life.

Bariatric patients speak of wanting to feel 'normal', to find the comforting anonymity of looking rather like everyone else. Weight loss allows people to feel confident about going out, visiting restaurants, theatres or cinemas, untroubled by the fear that they won't fit in the seats. They can book holidays and accept invitations to social events without worrying about being paralysed by self-consciousness. Weight loss following surgery often brings improvements in body image[39] and reduced distress about appearance. The change in your appearance after surgery can be very rapid and most people experience this cascading weight loss as highly motivating and exciting. However, for others the change in the image in the mirror can be unnerving – some people struggle to recognise themselves and need time to adjust to their new image.

Marriage and relationships

While people sometimes believe that weight loss surgery destabilises relationships, research evidence does not back this up. While your partner may need reassurance that losing weight won't lead you to seek another relationship, in general studies tend to find that most couples stay together after surgery and report greater relationship satisfaction,[40,41] and the small proportion of relationships that break down tend to be the ones where patients had spoken of marital or sexual problems before surgery.[42] As with all major challenges in life, the extent to which your relationship withstands the impact of weight loss surgery will depend upon the quality of the relationship and your ability to adapt and work together to make it a positive experience for the whole family. With improved health, social confidence and energy levels you may be able to return to activities that you enjoyed together in the past, such as dancing or going for long walks, so strengthening the relationship bond.

Hopefully the positive effects of surgery will rub off on your family. Weight loss surgery can be an opportunity for the people close to you to make healthy changes, becoming more active and modifying their diet.

> I have learnt so much about nutrition and I am ready to sort out my family's nutritional needs alongside my own.
>
> N, gastric bypass

Family members have been shown by some studies to experience a significant weight loss, with better eating habits, reduced emotional eating, increased activity levels and lower consumption of alcohol at 12 months after surgery. Even children of weight loss surgery patients appear to benefit with a normalisation of their weight.[43] Encouraging your partner to take on the new approach to healthy eating will be particularly important if he or she has a weight problem; one study found that spouses who are overweight are more likely to *gain* weight in the year following their partner's surgery,[44] perhaps because they are eating the leftovers!

Improved body confidence, a new sense of attractiveness and feeling more energetic, fewer problems with physical discomfort and increased confidence with personal hygiene, mean that many patients report an improvement in sexual relationships after surgery.[45] While half of weight loss surgery patients report some sexual difficulty before surgery, only 6 per cent do one year post-surgery[42] and both patients and their partners often rate themselves as enjoying sex more and having better orgasms after surgery.[46]

Reduced discrimination

Weight loss surgery patients report a dramatic decrease in their experience of discrimination after surgery.[47] A number of studies have shown that weight loss surgery can result in enhanced job prospects, better paid work, improved confidence in performing your job and greater likelihood of having personally satisfying work,[48] presumably due to a reduction in weight discrimination, improved self-esteem and mood, greater confidence and better health.

> I [got] . . . a better pay rise and more respect at work . . .
>
> A, gastric bypass

The virtuous cycle of weight loss, improved well-being and quality of life

As we saw in Chapter 3, obesity is associated with a range of physical and emotional problems that can have a severe impact on people's lives. Being severely overweight can lead to impairments in social and personal relationships, emotional well-being and self-esteem and reduced life choices. With the weight loss and improved health offered by weight loss surgery, many aspects of this vicious cycle can be reversed; patients report better mood, reduced shame and guilt, greater social confidence, they feel more energetic and face less discrimination. The impact of these positive changes can be seen in Figure 9.1, representing the virtuous cycle of weight loss.

Dealing with high risk situations

It's great news if you are doing well, losing weight and feeling healthy and optimistic. Your willpower feels invincible and you are determined to keep up all the positive changes you've made to your lifestyle. This is exactly the outcome that you and your bariatric team hoped for. Unfortunately willpower can weaken and our best intentions are tested by events in our lives that disrupt our routine or cause us to feel worried or unhappy. It is only human to find that you are being pulled back into old, less helpful patterns of behaviour.[49]

In Chapter 4 we heard about the stages of change model.[50] Once you have adapted to life after surgery, made changes to your eating

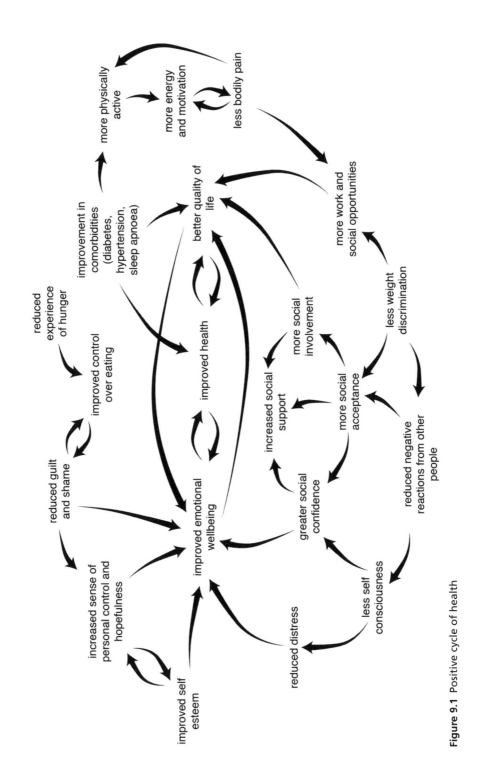

Figure 9.1 Positive cycle of health

habits and lifestyle, and achieved good weight loss, you are moving in the *maintenance* stage of the model. This stage is crucial in consolidating and strengthening the new behaviours you have put in place, but it's also a risky time. A change of job, the end of a relationship, the loss of a family member, ill health or financial difficulties can all swamp our coping resources and make it difficult to maintain positive change. Even a series of more minor hassles can make it hard for us to find the energy to keep up healthy behaviours. In this section we will consider some strategies that may be helpful to support your ongoing efforts or get you back on track if you have stumbled.

For anyone making changes to health behaviours and lifestyle there will be situations that are *high risk*;[51] those situations that cause you to feel less in control and make you vulnerable to going back to old behaviours. These may be internal factors, such as feeling sad, frustrated or bored; external situations, such as going on holiday, being alone in the house or work demands; or interpersonal situations, like conflict with family or friends. Social situations where there is overt or unspoken pressure to go back to unhelpful eating habits may also be high risk.

> [I'm more likely to eat the wrong things at] dinner parties where I am trying to be polite and eat what I am given.
>
> A, gastric bypass

Your response to these high risk situations will determine how confident you feel about maintaining positive change. Each time you successfully cope with a difficult situation it will heighten your feeling of *self-efficacy*. Self-efficacy is a personal sense of being able to do what needs to be done to reach a certain outcome[52] – in your case to eat well, stay active and achieve better health. High self-efficacy represents a belief that you have the coping skills to handle a particular situation. The greater your sense of mastery the more likely you are to treat a potentially difficult situation as a challenge and the more effort you will be able to put in to cope with obstacles or difficulties. If you don't have good self-efficacy in certain areas of life, your willingness to face problems head-on is diminished and you may seek to avoid the threat.

Each time you take on a difficult situation and cope, your sense of mastery and confidence grows. You can support your budding self-confidence by recognising danger points and having a clear idea about how you'll cope with them. Begin by asking yourself some questions:

- When am I most at risk of sliding back into old habits?
- What have I found useful in maintaining helpful behaviours?
- What changes have I already made in the way I think and behave?
- What have I found useful in controlling unhelpful behaviours?

- How can I make sure I continue to do these things?
- What barriers or blocks am I likely to face in maintaining these helpful behaviours in the future?
- How can I overcome these barriers?
- How will I know when I'm struggling? What will I notice in my behaviour? How will I feel? What might other people say to me?
- What will I do if I have a setback? Who will I ask to support me?

Use the answers to these questions as a roadmap to prepare for challenges and to guide your coping efforts. Think about the skills you already have that are helping you achieve the outcome you want and the skills you may still need to develop.

Challenge unhelpful thinking

Reflecting on the way you are viewing events in your life, standing back a little to give perspective and gently challenging unhelpful thoughts, can help you find a more useful way of thinking about things. It is not about being 'wrong' or 'stupid' and needing to think better; it's about being aware of how powerful emotions can draw your thinking in unhelpful directions and reduce your ability to cope effectively.

As we saw in Chapter 6, our 'old brain' uses emotions as a threat-protection system to alert us to threat, but our 'new brain' – our ability to think, reason and project into the future – can get caught up in this emotional wave causing us to ruminate on worries. You may experience high levels of self-critical thoughts; telling you that you should have done things better, that you should be a different kind of person, that you should feel or behave differently or be more able to cope. Challenging your thoughts in a compassionate way is not the same as self-criticism as it accepts that we all have weaknesses and failings and that we also have a wish to improve. Compassionate thought-balancing[53] emphasises growth, hopefulness and building on positives.

Different people can have very different emotional reactions to the same situation and this is reflected in their thinking about the event. Faced with a flat tyre on the motorway, Janet may remain quite calm. She thinks: 'It could be worse, at least I was able to pull over safely. Thank heavens I have my mobile so I can call the breakdown service. I'll have to wait a while but I'll get help.' Janet is able to hold on to the more reassuring aspects of her situation and trust that help will arrive. Sandra's thought is: 'I told John to check the tyres. It's not fair, it's going to cost me a fortune and I needed the money for Christmas.' She feels furious with her husband and panicky about the future. Louise feels distressed and helpless; the motorway breakdown feels like confirmation that everything always goes wrong for her: 'Why do these things always happen to me? I never make anything go right in my life. Everything is so hard.' This critical internal voice can generate painful feelings that are self-defeating; they reduce your confidence and prevent you from making good decisions.

Becoming aware of the nature of your thoughts, recognising that thoughts simply flow through the mind rather than representing a truthful reflection of reality, may feel a little strange at first, but the mindfulness exercises in Chapter 6 should help with the process. When you find yourself feeling anxious, upset or angry, step back from your thoughts and observe them. Attend to what is happening in your mind and try to 'catch' the significant thoughts amid the noise. It will be helpful to write them down and I have given an example of a thought-balancing diary below.

Remind yourself that whatever you are feeling is the way you are feeling and that is okay. Then, holding on to a feeling of kindness towards yourself, your thoughts and feelings, ask yourself the following series of questions:[53]

- Is this thinking helpful for me?
- Would I think like this if I wasn't upset? If I felt more relaxed or happier would I be seeing things differently?
- Are there other possible explanations for the situation other than the one that is making me feel sad, fearful or angry?
- Am I thinking about the world as if there are rigid rules about how things *should* be? Are rules about how life *should be* stopping me from thinking flexibly about this?
- Am I underestimating my ability to cope with this? What are my strengths? How have I used them to cope with difficulties in the past?
- Would I teach a child or friend to think like this? If not, how would I like them to think about these things? What would I say to a good friend in this situation? What would be helpful for someone else?
- How would I think about this at my compassionate best?

Using the answers to these questions you can build up a more helpful way of thinking about the situation. Focus on creating a warm, kind response – the sort you might get from your most compassionate friend. Don't worry initially about how much you *believe* the alternative response. You do not need to come up with entirely positive thoughts, this is not about pretending that everything is rosy and that difficult things don't happen in life.

By standing back from your thoughts and feelings, you can observe your thoughts and recognise old patterns of thinking and behaviour. You can become aware of anxious or angry thoughts and make a more balanced decision about how you will respond to them. Use this aware-ness to reflect on your thoughts, as if they are someone else's thoughts and feelings. See yourself as a concerned observer who wants the best

Table 9.1 Thought balancing diary

Gemma B–December 2010

DAY	TRIGGER SITUATION	UPSETTING THOUGHTS	COMPASSIONATE THOUGHT
Tues 10.15	Meeting a friend for coffee at the cafe, feeling anxious, unsettled and jittery.	'Susan will make a comment on my weight. I haven't lost as much as I should.'	'I haven't lost as much weight as I would like, which is frustrating but I have lost quite a bit and it's coming off steadily. I feel better in myself. I'm not failing, I just need to persevere.' 'I'm anticipating criticism and that's scary, but Susan is a good friend and I can trust her to be concerned for me.'
		'Why do I always fail at everything?' 'I want to cancel.'	'No one told me it would be easy and I knew it would be a challenge. I am working hard to get my eating under control and I need to have patience. I have shown patience before in my life and have survived some pretty difficult times.' 'My mind is telling me to run away, but I know that being with people makes me feel better in the long run. I learnt as a child not to trust people but now I want to be more courageous in asking for support.'
Fri 7 pm	Going out for dinner with friends. Feeling cross and worried.	'Everyone else will be able to eat what they want. Why do I have to be deprived?'	'No one likes to feel deprived and in the past I've found it almost unbearable but I've got better at tolerating these feelings. It's not helpful to me to compare myself with other people in these situations.'
		'I'll never feel normal.'	'So what's normal anyway? Everyone has their own problems to deal with. I have my own strengths and my own weaknesses and that's okay.'
		'I will lose control and eat too much.'	'In the past I've lost control of my eating especially if I felt sad or lonely. It helps if I'm kind to myself and eat slowly and mindfully.'

for you and who can provide valuable commentary on your emotional experience. So, for example, you may experience a wave of worry and loneliness when your husband is late home from work; use the compassionate thinking perspective to recognise and acknowledge the old pattern in your brain that is telling you to use food to calm yourself. Or another example might be when you are faced with a social event which is making you feel anxious, concerned that you will feel fat and self-conscious; try to accept your feelings of anxiety and note with interest and curiosity that your anxious mind is telling you to make an excuse and cancel.

Starting a thought-balancing diary

1. Pay careful attention to any difficult feelings you experience. In the second column, write down the situation you're in and the type of feelings – are you cross, frustrated, upset, sad, disappointed, furious?
2. Try to catch the upsetting thoughts that are swirling around in your mind. Write down these thoughts in the third column.
3. Use the questions above to create a more compassionate and helpful thought.
4. Next time you find yourself in a similar situation and the same upsetting thought is fixed in your mind, try to remember the kinder, more balanced response. If it's a frequent thought, write down the alternative thought and carry it with you in your purse or wallet as a reminder.

Remember, it helps a lot to write these thoughts down in a diary, rather than trying to work through the process in your mind. The act of writing down helps you recognise your efforts to change and offers a bit of perspective, some separation, from the emotional impact of the thought.

Coping with food cravings[54]

It is natural and normal to experience food cravings – an apparently irresistible urge to seek a particular kind of food. These cravings often have an emotional element and patients often speak about being 'addicted' to chocolate or cola, because these urges are so powerful. It is sometimes possible to create a space between the craving and your response to it, allowing you time to consider your choices.

Steinberg and Dryden (1996)[54] suggest that you ask yourself these questions when you experience a craving:

1. What am I craving?
2. What was happening just before I began to feel this craving?

3. What result can I expect if I give into temptation? How will I feel?
4. Is giving in to the urge the best or only way to handle it?
5. Would some alternative activity satisfy or distract me?
6. Which do I choose this time: immediate gratification or mild frustration in exchange for long-term success?

They suggest that, if you decide on immediate gratification, you make an agreement with yourself that you will still do an alternative activity for 15 minutes first. I would add that if, after this 15 minutes, you still decide to act on the craving that you do so mindfully – take the food to the table and eat it slowly and with full consciousness.

Think about consequences

When people have a desire to do something, such as eat a particular food or drink too much alcohol, they tend to emphasise the positives and ignore the negatives. So for example, people are likely to drink more alcohol if they have a strong expectation of positive outcomes, like having fun, being sociable or feeling more confident, and downplay the negative outcomes, such as having a hangover, embarrassing themselves or making themselves ill. If you are tempted to eat the kinds of foods that will get in the way of your long-term goal, ask yourself what the *positive* consequences will be. You may note that you anticipate feelings of pleasure or that it will ease feelings of stress. Now acknowledge the *negative* consequences – it may be that you will feel guilty afterwards or that the choice confirms damaging self-beliefs; it could lead to some loss of control of eating or leave you to feeling physically uncomfortable. Before you make your decision reflect on these advantages and disadvantages – at the very least it will give you a moment of pause to think about your actions.

Avoid turning a lapse into a relapse

If you encounter a problem in a high risk situation and experience a lapse in your best intentions, try to avoid blaming it on a character flaw. If you say to yourself 'I have no willpower, I'll never be able to change!' you are effectively deciding that you will never be able to cope in that situation and that will have a knock-on effect on your confidence in a whole range of difficult situations. Instead, acknowledge your human frailty and make a mental note that you need to develop some more effective coping strategies for that situation, be it going to a friend's house for dinner or facing a Sunday evening on your own. Allow yourself to learn from your mistakes rather than beating yourself up about them.

Summary

As you can see from this chapter many patients experience profound improvements in their health, emotional well-being and quality of life following surgery. These patients often describe surgery as the best thing they ever did. When successful, surgery can produce life-changing weight loss, resolve life-threatening illness, increase life expectancy, allow people to feel happier, more confident and offer new opportunities and life choices.

Even those people who do very well with surgery will face challenges and it helps to identify your potential high risk situations. Develop a plan or road map of how you will manage these challenges and think out the coping skills and support you'll need at these times. Use a thought diary to develop compassionate thinking skills to help dissipate self-critical and unhelpful thoughts. Work on your skills in coping with the inevitable food cravings. Take a pause before making a potentially unhelpful decision, to give yourself a chance to reflect on the consequences, but if you do have a slip-up try to avoid blaming set-backs on weaknesses in your personality as this tends to detract from positive coping and makes you more vulnerable to relapse.

10

'I thought if I was slim the world would be some kind of fairy tale': the risks and challenges of weight loss surgery

If you're thinking about weight loss surgery, hoping it is the permanent answer to your weight problem, you may be reluctant to read about the things that go wrong. It can feel easier to turn your head away from potential risks and complications, to focus instead on thoughts of the great life you'll have when you've lost loads of weight. Nevertheless, I would encourage you not to skip this chapter; weight loss surgery is a profoundly life-changing event – often for the better, but sometimes for the worse.

> Each time [surgeons] perform our bariatric surgery, we are doing it with the hope and expectation of excellent weight loss, patient relief from comorbidities, no complications, short-term hospital stay, as well as ample satisfaction and compliance from each of our patients . . . Yet, those of us who perform any numbers of this surgery know that we will experience, at some time or other, a leak, poor weight loss, some refractory comorbidities, prolonged hospital stay [and] malignant non-compliance.
>
> Cowan 1998: 77[1]

When I talk about the risks of weight loss surgery, many people say to me: 'Yes, but I could get knocked down by a bus tomorrow,' but of course getting hit by a bus is not something that we would request and plan for. We all need to take some risks in order to lead a full life and you may feel that weight loss surgery is a risk worth taking, but you still need to know what can go wrong. You owe it to yourself, and your family and friends, to know as much as you can about the problems you may face after surgery for a number of reasons. First, you cannot make a balanced decision about surgery without weighing the potential benefits against the possible risks. Second, some problems are preventable and knowing the pitfalls may help you avoid them. Finally, some medical and psychological complications can be very severe, even life-threatening; you must be able to recognise whether the problem you're experiencing is normal and benign, or whether you need to seek immediate help and advice from your bariatric team.

In this chapter we will look at the surgical complications associated with weight loss surgery as well as the ongoing social and emotional challenges some people face in the months and years after surgery. If you have already had surgery, take some time to go through the post-surgery MOT test at the end of the chapter to review progress and highlight any areas that you need to work on. You can use this checklist to review your progress regularly in the months following surgery.

Medical and surgical complications

Risk of death

While weight loss surgery is now broadly considered an effective and reasonably safe treatment for obesity, it is not without risks. For understandable reasons the risk patients are often most concerned about (though less common than other surgical or medical complications) is the risk of death (the *mortality rate*).

Mortality rates have reduced over the years due to improvements in surgical techniques, the establishment of specialist centres and surgical training programmes and increased monitoring. Nowadays, it is thought that between one and three per thousand patients die within 30 days of having a bariatric procedure.[2,3,4,5] The mortality rate is rather lower for gastric band at around one per 2,000 patients and higher with the sleeve gastrectomy (at around one to two people per 500[6]) and gastric bypass, but are greater if you need *open* surgery.[2,3,7] The most common causes of death in the month following surgery are sepsis following a leak (33 per cent), a cardiac event (28 per cent) and pulmonary embolism (17 per cent).[5] For 12-month mortality for gastric bypass and sleeve, NHS advice gives a broad figure of 1 per cent. These mortality rates are based on results from specialist bariatric centres. Where surgeons are less experienced or the centre only does a relatively low number of bariatric procedures each year, the mortality and complication rates might be higher.

The higher mortality rates for sleeve gastrectomy, gastric bypass and biliopancreatic diversion/duodenal switch (BPD/DS) patients reflect the greater surgical complexity and also the fact that these patients tend to have a higher body weight and more health problems. The risk of death is not equal across all weight loss surgery patients. Men are more at risk, as are people with a BMI over 50; older patients; those with a history of coronary artery disease, high blood pressure, deep vein thrombosis, pulmonary embolism and breathing problems, such as sleep apnoea or hypoventilation.[8,9] If you are considered too high risk for surgery, you may be offered an interim procedure, such as a gastric balloon, to bring your weight down.[10]

Complications

The likelihood of developing complications depends upon your health and body weight before surgery, as well as the type of bariatric procedure and your ability to stick to the rules about how and what to eat after surgery. When making a decision about weight loss surgery it's important you are fully aware of the problems you potentially face, even if you believe the likely benefits are definitely worth the risk.

Broadly speaking the risks, in terms of death rates, having to use open (rather than keyhole) surgery, serious complications and need for re-admission, are somewhat higher for the gastric bypass than the sleeve gastrectomy and the risks of the sleeve are somewhat higher than the gastric band.[3] The most common serious problems immediately after surgery are anastomotic leak, internal bleeding and pulmonary embolism.[11] The risks associated with the gastric bypass, sleeve gastrectomy and biliopancreatic diversion with duodenal switch are greater than for the gastric band as they are longer and more complex procedures. Men with a BMI over 50; older patients and those with a history of coronary artery disease, high blood pressure, deep vein thrombosis, pulmonary embolism and breathing problems are at greater risk of being re-admitted to hospital, developing deep vein thrombosis (DVT) and needing blood transfusion.[12]

A proportion of all bariatric patients will need revisional surgery to correct or reverse the initial procedure or to convert to another type of procedure where the original operation has failed. Revisional surgery carries an increased risk of complications and death and should only be undertaken in specialist centres where the surgeon has extensive experience.[13]

General complications of abdominal surgery

There are a number of surgical complications that are seen with all abdominal surgery, rather than being specific to bariatric surgery. These include internal bleeding, cardiovascular problems, infection and the development of hernias.

Bleeding

Bleeding into the abdomen or bowel may occur within a few hours of surgery; 3–5 per cent of bariatric patients experience post-surgical bleeding, requiring blood transfusion or surgery.[14]

Cardiovascular complications

Cardiovascular complications include myocardial infarction, stroke, pulmonary embolism, DVT and cardiac arrest. Surgery and reduced activity increase the likelihood of blood clotting. Blood clots formed in the legs are known as DVT. If this blood clot breaks off and moves to the lungs it is called a pulmonary embolus (PE) and is potentially life-threatening. The risk can be reduced by wearing compression stockings while in hospital and you will be encouraged to get up and walking as soon as possible after surgery. You may also be prescribed blood thinning medication, like heparin. The rates of cardiovascular complications range from one person per 500 for gastric band to one person in a 100 for sleeve gastrectomy.[2]

Infection

After surgery people can develop chest or urinary tract infections or infections at the wound site and need treatment with antibiotics. The risk of lung infection is reduced by carrying out breathing exercises as advised by the physiotherapist post-surgery.

Hernia

Incisional hernias, a bulge that develops at the surgical incision, are rare with laparoscopic surgery, but are a common complication of open surgery. Internal hernias, an abnormal opening in the stomach pouch, can potentially cause blockage of the bowel.

Injury to the spleen

Inadvertent injury to the spleen during surgery is rare, but in some cases can result in having the spleen removed, which has lifelong implications for immune function.

Complications specific to bariatric surgery[3]

Leakage

Leaks can occur along the staple line or where the small intestine is joined to the stomach pouch (*anastomotic leak*). Between one and six people in 200 gastric bypass, sleeve gastrectomy and BPD/DS patients experience leakage from the gastrointestinal tract if a full seal does not form where the stomach and intestine are joined. Leakage can be a particular problem with the sleeve gastrectomy because of technical surgical reasons.

The leak allows the stomach or bowel contents to enter the abdominal cavity leading to serious infection and possibly sepsis. Sepsis is an extreme response to infection where the body releases chemicals and hormones causing inflammation which then affects the entire body, potentially leading to organ failure and death. Symptoms can include a rapid heart rate, fast breathing and fever. Some leaks can be treated with antibiotics but most will require immediate re-operation.

Gastrocutaneous fistulae, where there is a space linking the stomach to the skin resulting in severe infection or sepsis, is a rare but again potentially life-threatening complication of bariatric surgery.[15]

Intestinal obstruction

Obstruction of the intestine can be caused by abdominal scar tissue (adhesions), an internal hernia or severe constipation. Just over 1 per cent of gastric bypass patients have a problem with obstruction[16] with symptoms of nausea, abdominal bloating, vomiting and abdominal pain, and most will need a further operation to resolve the problem.

Stricture

Anastomotic stricture happens when there is a tightening of the hole between the stomach pouch and the small intestine, due to natural constriction of the join as it heals, preventing the swallowing of food and fluids. It can usually be managed by an endoscopic procedure in which a balloon is inflated to open up the hole.

Ulcers

Ulcers are sores that occur in the stomach pouch or around the new join of the stomach pouch and small intestine due to a restricted blood supply. Symptoms can include pain or burning sensation in the upper abdomen, vomiting or difficulty tolerating certain foods.

Smoking increases the risk of ulcers and you will need to avoid certain medications, especially non-steroidal, anti-inflammatory drugs (NSAIDs), including aspirin and ibuprofen. Other pills may need to be crushed or taken in liquid form; ask your bariatric team or doctor if you are unsure which medications to use.

Gastrogastric fistula

A gastrogastric fistula is an opening that develops between the gastric pouch and the remnant stomach. It results in impaired restriction, allowing people to eat high volumes of food without satiety, and so results in poor weight loss. It is associated with ulcers developing in the stomach pouch.

Gallstone disease

A relatively high proportion of number of gastric bypass and BPD/DS patients develop gallstone disease due to rapid weight loss and need to have their gallbladder removed (known as a *cholescystectomy*). Some surgeons feel it is best routinely to remove the gallbladder at the same time as performing the gastric bypass surgery.[17]

Complications with the gastric band

The key surgical complications that occur with gastric band are band slippage and erosion[11,18] with 10–20 per cent of band patients needing a further operation.[19] Band slippage occurs when the band becomes misplaced, with a part of the stomach moving up through the band to create a larger upper stomach pouch, possibly due to frequent vomiting or overeating. Symptoms of slippage include upper abdominal pain, acid reflux, vomiting and problems eating. Investigation is by x-ray and the band is deflated. The surgeon then has to make a decision as to whether the band can be repositioned and stitched into place or whether it needs to be removed. Erosion, affecting about 4 per cent of patients, occurs when the band cuts into the wall of the stomach and always requires the removal of the band.[11] You may not have any symptoms or you may experience general abdominal pain, nausea or problems tolerating solid foods.

Pouch dilation, stretching of the stomach pouch, is usually the result of overeating and is indicated by a reduced sense of fullness when you eat and possibly some reflux symptoms. Dilation of the oesophagus is a relatively rare complication, characterised by increasing problems with swallowing, vomiting and chest pain, again requiring removal of the band.

The band can be become blocked if you eat without sufficient care, especially difficult to chew foods like foods such as bread, pasta, the skins of fruit or red meat. Blockage causes discomfort, vomiting and inability to eat or drink, and may require a trip to hospital to have the band loosened. Leakage of fluid from the band or band tubing results in loss of restriction, ability to eat more without feeling full, increased tolerance for a range of foods and weight regain. The port used for band fills can become infected, or may twist requiring a minor procedure to reposition it.

A proportion of gastric band patients require conversion to the gastric bypass or sleeve gastrectomy because of inadequate weight loss or complications. The average hospital stay after this revisional surgery is two to four days and patients achieve an average weight loss of 41 per cent of excess weight over two years.[20]

Ongoing difficulties following weight loss surgery

If you are careful about following dietary guidelines, you should not experience too many problems and side effects such as diarrhoea, constipation, difficulty swallowing, vomiting and flatulence generally reduce over the months after surgery. However some people find that they continue to experience ongoing problems with discomfort, vomiting or diarrhoea that affect their physical and emotional well-being. If this occurs your first response should be to review how and what you're eating. Are you eating foods that are suitable for your stage? Are you taking your time to eat carefully? Are you eating or drinking too quickly? Are you trying to eat solid, textured foods too soon after surgery? Are you trying to eat too much? If you are experiencing serious pain or discomfort or are feeling unwell or feverish, you should contact your bariatric team immediately.

Vomiting

Vomiting is a common effect of weight loss surgery as you adapt to living with a smaller stomach pouch. Up to two-thirds of patients experience vomiting after surgery, mostly in the months following surgery, but for some continuing for years.[21] Ongoing frequent vomiting can be due to medical complications, such as intestinal obstruction, anastomotic stricture, ulcers or blockage of a gastric band, but most commonly is in response to poorly chewed food, inappropriate food choices, mixing drinks with foods or the consumption of overly large portions. To reduce vomiting you need to eat slowly, taking small bites, avoiding tough foods that are difficult to chew to a paste.[22] Vomiting can also be caused by dehydration so ensure that you drink plenty of fluids.

Persistent vomiting can lead to nutritional deficiencies and complications. If you're vomiting frequently despite making changes to your diet and eating habits, you may need to be investigated for stricture or intestinal obstruction. If you have a gastric band this may need to be loosened.

Dumping syndrome

Dumping syndrome occurs in around 50–70 per cent of gastric bypass patients.[23] It is caused by eating sugary foods which trigger changes in blood sugar and insulin levels, causing symptoms such as nausea, vomiting, palpitations, weakness, sweating, stomach cramps, faintness and diarrhoea. The experience of dumping can be very unpleasant and may leave you feeling washed out and exhausted for a number of hours, however bariatric surgeons and dietitians view it as a useful learning experience, training patients not to consume sugary, high calorie foods.

> [If I'm having a meal out] my fear of dumping syndrome makes me select food carefully . . . I don't want to collapse in public!
>
> N, gastric bypass

You can minimise the problem of dumping[2] by:

- Increasing your consumption of protein.
- Limiting how much sugary food, such as chocolate, sweets, cake and biscuits, you eat. Look out for high levels of glucose, fructose, dextrose, all of which are simply different forms of sugar, on food labels.
- Eating more complex carbohydrates, such as wholegrain foods, which take longer to digest.
- Avoiding high sugar drinks such as milkshakes, hot chocolate, fruit juice and sweet tea or coffee. Instead have low sugar drinks such as sugar-free squash.
- Have more frequent small meals a day rather than three large meals.
- Eat slowly and avoid drinking until 20 minutes after your meal.

> I don't cheat at all, as it can lead to the dumping syndrome which is nasty; I look at the back of every packet when we shop, in case anything has hidden sugars or fats. It is amazing how many things we think are healthy are actually not.
>
> K, gastric bypass

Food intolerance

> It's a shock when Oxo is your only food source.
>
> J, gastric bypass

Some people find there are a number of foods that they can't tolerate after surgery. Starchy foods, such as bread, pasta and rice, and fibrous foods like red meat, sweet corn, celery, tomato skins and pineapple, can be a problem, potentially causing stomach pain and bloating.

> [I sometimes make myself unwell] . . . usually from eating too much of a food or trying something I hadn't recently. Like most pork

makes me sick, or too much meat . . . Also if I eat too much rice or pasta.

> A, gastric bypass

[I get] sickness, especially with certain foods – mine is bread, eggs and milk at the moment.

> J, gastric bypass

If you've have a gastric band the bariatric team will be trying to find the 'sweet spot' where the band offers you restriction and you lose weight steadily, but not so tight that you find it difficult to tolerate any foods and are vomiting frequently. The band is *too loose* if you are able to eat large portions of solid crunchy foods; you are getting hungry and snacking during the day; and are showing no weight loss or weight gain. The band is *too tight* if you are only able to eat soft foods or liquids; food gets struck and won't go through the band leading to vomiting; you frequently experience heartburn; you are losing weight rapidly or gaining weight because you are relying on high calorie drinks. The band fill is about right if you are able to eat solid crunchy foods; are satisfied with small portions; are not hungry or snacking between meals; and are losing ½ –1kg a week.[24] If you feel your band is too tight or too loose you need to contact your bariatric team.

Not being able to eat certain foods can lead to unhealthy choices, including an over-reliance on soft, sweet foods[25] which will make it much harder for you to achieve good weight loss.

I couldn't eat bread, I couldn't eat rice, I couldn't eat meat. I couldn't eat any fruit or vegetables . . . I ate custard, yoghurts, rice pudding, sweet stuff . . . I could eat biscuits, cake chocolate . . . anything that was sweet.

> Weight loss surgery patient who had experienced weight regain quoted in Ogden *et al.* 2006: 284[25]

There have been reports of bariatric patients developing a problem with eating non-food substances, such as ice, though this seems to be more common in patients who have previously had a problem with this type of disordered eating.[26]

Nutritional deficiencies

Surgery that restricts the absorption of calories and nutrients from the food you eat, most particularly BPD/DS but also gastric bypass, can result in nutritional complications, including protein malnutrition and deficiencies in iron, folate, calcium, zinc, B vitamins and fat-soluble vitamins (A, K, E and D). Nutritional deficiencies are more likely to occur if you are vomiting frequently or if you are unable to take in adequate amounts of food and are losing weight rapidly.

[. . .] five months after surgery my hair started to fall out by the brush-full, it got very thin in amount and texture. My fingernails split and broke. The [support] group told me to take . . . extra vitamins and eat more protein which I did and it has now started to recover. This was a very scary time for me . . . 'thin but bald' was not what I had signed up for.

J, sleeve gastrectomy

Nutritional deficiencies can be avoided by ensuring that you have a balanced, nutritious diet and take vitamin and mineral supplements regularly, but if they do occur they can result in hair loss, fatigue, loss of muscle, headaches, palpitations, loss of night vision and depression.[22] Your bariatric team may suggest you use protein supplements and may offer vitamin B^{12} injections.

In rare cases, biliopancreatic diversion and gastric bypass patients have developed *Wernicke's encephalopathy*, a type of brain damage, due to vitamin B^1 (thiamine) deficiency.[27] Increased risk of Wernicke's encephalopathy is associated with excessive weight loss, frequent vomiting, malabsorption of vitamins and alcohol abuse.[28] The symptoms are confusion, loss of muscle coordination, abnormal eye movements and double vision. Treatment with thiamine injections can prevent symptoms from worsening, but almost half of these patients will continue to experience some residual problems with memory, walking and coordination difficulties after treatment.[29]

Acid reflux

Very overweight people often suffer from reflux disease, where acid from the stomach comes up into the oesophagus causing symptoms of heartburn. In many cases this is resolved with weight loss after surgery, but some patients develop or continue to experience symptoms post-surgery.

Emotional and behavioural problems after surgery

I thought if I was slim the world would be some kind of fairy tale.

Sarah, who lost 6st through dieting,
quoted in *Times Magazine*, p30[30]

As we have seen in Chapter 3, obesity has a profound impact on emotional and social well-being and for most bariatric patients the experience of dramatic weight loss enables them to feel more positive, socially confident and active. However, the restriction of food can lead to emotional strain, particularly for those people who have used food to manage difficult feelings. The sheer speed of weight loss can also be unnerving and adjusting to your new place in the world poses some often overlooked challenges. For some the rapid weight loss creates feelings of vulnerability, with increased anxiety about attention from others or fear of illness.

Deterioration in mental health

> [My emotional health] has actually gotten much worse because you
> constantly step on scales, beat yourself up if you have not lost
> weight or made a bad food choice, sometimes feel like everyone
> stares at you MORE then when you were large because now you are
> a funny shape. Before I KNEW I could not find clothes that fit, now
> I think, 'Oh that should fit' but in every shop I am a different size,
> sometimes much larger, sometimes much smaller and everything
> for me is now out of proportion so it is upsetting and stressful.
>
> A, gastric bypass

A number of studies have shown that being depressed or anxious before surgery does not in itself have an impact on weight loss[31] and most patients report an improvement in their mood after surgery. However this is likely to depend to a large extent on the original reason for the emotional difficulties. Where a person has been depressed or anxious because of their weight and its effect on their quality of life or social relationships, it's likely that their emotional state will improve as they lose weight. However, where the mental health difficulties are unrelated to obesity, the surgery may offer little benefit to emotional well-being or indeed could cause a serious deterioration in emotional health.

The removal of food as a source of pleasure or comfort can present an emotional challenge for people with a history of emotional eating – using food to suppress or distract from difficult feelings. As almost half of bariatric patients describe themselves as emotional eaters[32] it's not surprising that some patients find that the emotional strain of surgery is far greater than they had imagined.

> [After surgery] I was probably slightly more emotional and did get
> angry easier, which ultimately did lead to being treated for anxiety
> and depression.
>
> A, gastric bypass

People with a history of severe mental health difficulties, such as psychotic disorders, bipolar disorder, major depression or personality disorders are at risk of experiencing a relapse of their illness as they face the strain of coping with surgery and the changes to their lifestyle even despite good weight loss.[33] These patients may struggle to accept support from others and have difficulty with taking sufficient care of their health and dietary needs after surgery. Research suggests that people with a history of hospitalisation for psychiatric care, who have an untreated personality disorder, or multiple psychiatric diagnoses are at greater risk of medical complications and psychological disturbance following surgery.[34,35] Studies have found that there is an increased risk of weight loss surgery patients needing admission into psychiatric care[36] and the incidence of suicide is greater in bariatric patients than the general public.[37,38] One bariatric professional commented rather bluntly on the risk of deterioration in mood and increased suicide rate among weight loss surgery patients:

> This happens when the wrong people are having surgery
> without the appropriate steps (such as counselling) in place. If
> they think their life is s**t because they're fat and they lose it and
> realise their life is still s**t for other reasons, it can tip them over
> the edge.
>
> *Times Magazine*, p29 [30]

Reports also exist of weight loss surgery patients replacing one *addiction* for another after surgery[39] as they are no longer able to use food as a means to regulate difficult emotions. This has been termed *addiction transfer* and may be in the form of an emergence or exacerbation of drug or alcohol use, or behavioural problems such as gambling or compulsive sex. Excessive preoccupation with shopping, computer games or social networking sites may also reflect a compulsive need to escape or block out feelings where previously food was used.

> [Weight loss surgery was not successful] because I am not scared of
> it and tested my boundaries. And what can I say, I eat within my
> limits but I DO love food . . . and I like alcohol. Too many patients
> do not recognize or acknowledge addiction transfer and I know
> many women who transfer their eating habits onto alcohol,
> shopping etc which can be just as damaging to your life as being
> large.
>
> A, gastric bypass

> I did start to substitute alcohol for food. But that became worse
> later on . . .I became an alcoholic . . . it was easier and easier to
> drink to fulfil the need in me
>
> Gastric bypass patient quoted in Ogden *et al.* 2011: 957 [40]

Change in relationships and friendships

Most people describe improved relationships after surgery; patients often feel more confident, self-assured and outgoing and are able to join in activities with family or friends that they previously found difficult. However, this new-found lease of life can also cause challenges, disrupting the dynamics of a relationship. The experience of feeling energetic and confident, with more time spent socialising or in new hobbies and interests can be interpreted by insecure partners as a 'change in personality'.[41]

Some patients feel glad, even euphoric, as others begin to see them differently, but at the same time may question whether their partner is fulfilling their emotional, social or sexual needs. They may feel drawn to seek other opportunities, potentially with an increase in risky contacts or behaviours. The experience of being found sexually desirable can rock an established relationship if the patient tests out their new sexual power. Your change in appearance could also lead to a fracture in a relationship if, for example, your partner's sexual preference is primarily for very large people.

Partners and friends may feel alienated by the changes they see happening in you or undermined by your new image.

> I started getting fewer and fewer calls [from friends]. I still keep asking a really good friend of mine about meeting up, but it's been a year now. She knew me at my biggest and she's big too. I think she just doesn't want to see me slim, so she fobs me off. I'd probably feel the same if I were in her situation.
>
> Lizzie Lee, gastric bypass patient, quoted in
> *Times Magazine*, p29 [30]

If your partner, friends or family are more sedentary, they might feel resentful or neglected as a result of your new routine; increased assertiveness can be perceived by others as selfishness; and a new enthusiasm for the world can feel threatening to those around you. Some husbands have described their wives as becoming 'excessively sociable' after surgery.[41]

Other weight loss surgery patients don't feel they can be honest about how they've lost weight, fearing criticism from others. Concern about being judged and a personal sense of having somehow failed may cause you to feel distanced from other people and less able to seek support.

> I don't want people to judge. I don't want people to think I've cheated. I feel a failure about it – I didn't do it of my own accord.
>
> Lizzie Lee, quoted in *Times Magazine,* p29 [30]

People may also resent your new eating habits, particularly if you acted as *food buddy* to your partner, best friend or sister – normalising the consumption of large amounts of food and spreading the guilt.[41] Your old partner in crime may feel left behind, abandoned or envious and you may need to work hard to find another focus for the time you spend together.

On the other hand the people around you may simply struggle to understand the changes you're trying to make and inadvertently make things just a little harder:

> [People] just always questioning what I am doing, how I am doing it, should I be doing it . . . People forget you are an adult and can make informed choices on what you eat, how you exercise, what feels and is right for body, stomach and mind . . .
>
> A, gastric bypass

Increased attention

Patients are often struck by the wave of compliments they receive as they're losing weight and this can lead some to feel uncomfortable and self-conscious. This positive feedback can also highlight a sense that they were viewed negatively before surgery.[42]

> You are invisible when you're big, even though there's more of you. When I'm at work there are a couple of [men] who always offer me a tea and make an effort to talk now. I think, well, you never made me a drink when I was big. It upsets me because I'm still the same person on the inside. It hurts to think that people don't want to know you as a person; they're just interested in the packaging.
>
> Sarah, quoted in *Times Magazine*, p30 [30]

Although most weight loss surgery patients report feeling more self-assured in social situations, and less worried about facing discrimination or abuse from others, some continue to feel anxious about other people's reactions. Somewhat counter-intuitively, patients who lose more weight after surgery seem more likely to experience a fear of negative judgements compared to those who lose less weight. When patients do continue to experience this self-consciousness and fear of negative reactions, it is associated with higher levels of depression and lowered quality of life.[43]

Complimentary remarks about your appearance may feel intrusive or sexually charged. Increased sexual attention from other people may feel threatening, embarrassing or simply confusing.

> I went into a bit of a shell to lose all this weight, then I came out the other side and found the world treats you differently . . . I never

clocked [the way men check women out] before, and it made me
paranoid. I felt too much attention on me; I felt too obvious.

Sarah, quoted in *Times Magazine,* p30 [30]

Feelings of vulnerability caused by this new attention may be
particularly pronounced for those patients with a history of abuse,
where the weight may have acted as a form of defence from sexual or
intimate relationships, or those who have little experience of dating and
relationships. Most studies have found no difference between people
who suffered sexual abuse and others in terms of weight loss, but victims
of abuse do seem to be more vulnerable to emotional difficulties after
weight loss surgery. This emotional disturbance may be considerable
and one study found that people with history of sexual abuse have a
greater risk of requiring psychiatric hospitalisation after surgery.[44]

Inadequate weight loss, weight regain and problematic eating

Some patients simply do not do well with surgery, losing minimal
weight or starting to regain weight after only a few months post-
surgery. Most studies have found that poor weight loss or excessive
weight regain is due to poor compliance with the post-surgery dietary
guidelines, in particular where this is associated with a re-emergence
of uncontrolled eating.

Poor weight loss

Around 20 per cent of patients fail to reach to best weight loss or begin
to regain weight too soon after surgery.[23] This is almost always associated with a difficulty in following the postoperative diet, with some
people increasing their calorie consumption significantly.[45] There is no
magic in bariatric surgery that prevents you from consuming too many
calories. Some studies suggest that up to a third of weight loss surgery
patients are unable or unwilling to comply with the recommended
dietary and lifestyle changes, by continuing to snack[46], using drinks to
wash down food so they can eat more, or consuming too much alcohol[47]
and these behaviours are evident in patients whose weight loss
plateaus early, by 12 months post-surgery.[48]

Other patients eat less food, but continue to take the same high
proportion of overall calories from fat as before surgery.[46] Often people
want gastric bypass because they see dumping syndrome as the
solution to their craving for sweet foods. They believe that they won't
'get away with' eating chocolate or ice cream. However a significant
minority of patients don't experience dumping. Others experience
minimal restriction on their food intake after surgery or still feel
significant hunger. As there is little to stop them eating as much as

they were before surgery or consuming high calorie food and drink, these patients are likely to have less than optimal weight loss.

> It's a physical pain in your stomach if you don't eat, it just makes me feel sicker and sicker and . . . you know what it's like to be sick with hunger
>
> Gastric band patient quoted in Ogden *et al.* 2005: 271 [49]

Poor weight loss has been linked to total calorie consumption; higher subjective hunger; dissatisfaction with appearance; increased tolerance for large amounts of food due to adapting to feelings of fullness; grazing; and continued emotional eating.[40,50,51] Relying on surgery to provide 'enough' restriction and so control food intake completely, or alternatively testing boundaries or trying to 'cheat' the restrictions, rather than working with the surgery and taking personal responsibility for your choices, will mean that you don't achieve the best weight loss.

Weight regain

> When Sue began to put on some weight, she started to feel helpless and panicky; her mealtime routines disappeared and her eating became erratic. She became caught in a vicious spiral of weight regain.

Bariatric surgery is often promoted as a permanent solution to obesity and many people are unaware of the likelihood of weight regain in the years following surgery. Some weight regain is normal; with gastric bypass there is average weight regain of 10–15 per cent of previously lost weight, usually starting around two years. However, a proportion of patients experience problematic weight gain, with almost 1 in 10 gastric bypass patients and a quarter of gastric band patients back to within 5 per cent of their pre-surgery weight at ten years follow-up.[45]

> My main fear now is that I [will] stretch my pouch and then eat too much.
>
> N, gastric bypass

Factors related to weight regain seem to be having a large proportion of high calorie foods in the diet; snacking through the day; eating in response to stress or upset; changes in physical or mental health that affect your ability to maintain the necessary lifestyle changes including regular exercise; altered metabolic rate as the result of illness, medication or age; and reduced self-monitoring of diet and exercise.[51] One study showed, perhaps predictably, that weight regain in the years following bypass was greatest in those patients who reported episodes of loss of control of their eating.[52]

A return to problematic eating

While most people report better control over their eating after surgery, there is growing evidence that some weight loss surgery patients struggle to stick to the post-surgery dietary advice and may revert to old eating habits. This may occur as the surgical restriction diminishes or when you learn how to get around the restriction by having high calorie drinks or snacking on small amounts throughout the day (a pattern of eating called grazing). Patients who had disordered eating habits before surgery often describe episodes of loss of control over their eating continuing after surgery, with grazing replacing binge episodes.[53] Though unable to consume the very large amounts of food after surgery that would constitute a binge episode, nevertheless some people continue to eat to the point of feeling uncomfortably full or vomiting and this is likely to result in poor weight loss.[54]

> I thought surgery would be it, I thought it would be a magic wand, but it is possible to cheat a bypass. I eat lots of crisps . . . I graze.
>
> Lizzie Lee, quoted in *Times Magazine*, p29[30]

Of patients with a diagnosis of binge eating disorder before surgery, 60 per cent describe grazing and some loss of control of their eating after surgery. This study by Colles *et al.* (2008)[50] found poor eating control to be associated with higher calorie intake, a greater proportion of fat in the diet, elevated feelings of hunger, a lower sense of being able to resist food, difficulty responding to satiety (full) signals, more symptoms of vomiting and lesser weight loss.

> I would have Chinese [takeaway] half, well quarter, of the Chinese at night, I'd get up in the middle of the night and have some more and then I would get up and have the rest probably for breakfast.
>
> Gastric band patient quoted in Ogden *et al.* 2011: 955 [40]

Uncontrolled eating is often triggered by distress and these patients report more depression and poorer emotional well-being. People who have always used food to relieve feelings of upset, anger, anxiety or aloneness are at risk of poor weight loss, and the more severe the pre-surgery emotional eating, the less weight loss you are likely to achieve.[55,56] There has been a suggestion that these at-risk patients are more often young women who report dissatisfaction with their appearance[50] but any bariatric patient with a history of disordered or emotional eating may have challenges in this area.

> I've been aware that food has become an emotional crutch, if you like . . . I eat my emotions . . .
>
> Gastric band patient quoted in Ogden *et al.* 2011: 956 [40]

> Triggers [for overeating] are normally someone telling me I should not eat something or that I am not 'behaving' but also if I get really low with my depression.
>
> A, gastric bypass

If you have a history of gaining weight at times of high personal stress; you have become upset as a result of trying to restrict your eating during a diet; or if you have times when you 'eat and eat' and struggle to stop, you may be particularly at risk of difficulties with the control of your eating after surgery. If you know you are an emotional eater it may be wise to resolve this behaviour before surgery; you need to feel confident in your ability to use other strategies to cope with difficult feelings to prevent this from derailing your efforts after surgery. It is possible to change emotional eating habits, but it will require some hard work and persistence and it may be appropriate to seek professional support. There's information about self-help resources and useful organisations in Chapter 11 and you can also look back over the ideas in Chapter 6.

Post-surgical eating avoidance

It is normal for rapid weight loss, however much desired, to be unsettling. It affects your self-image and the way others relate to you, requiring you to adjust to a new place in your social world. The experience of the changes in your body and the mismatch between expectation and reality can be disquieting.

> [After the initial euphoria] it's like your new body isn't your body. It's not been your body for such a long time . . . I thought if I was slim the world would be some kind of fairytale. But losing weight bought a whole new set of problems.
>
> Sarah, quoted in *Times Magazine*, p30 [30]

Some weight loss surgery patients become increasingly distressed about their appearance and preoccupied with losing more and more weight. There have been cases reported where patients develop an eating disorder similar to anorexia or bulimia. These patients develop an intense fear of weight regain and experience distress even thinking about the prospect of a weight increase. They have a distorted body image and use excessive food restriction or vomiting to prevent weight gain. This collection of characteristic behaviours and anxieties has been termed *post-surgical eating avoidance*[57] and is associated with rapid weight loss, non-compliance with dietary guidelines, avoidance of appointments, denial of a problem and high levels of anxiety. Some of these patients may also have bulimic episodes where they compensate for overeating through self-induced vomiting or try to assuage hunger by chewing on non-foods, such as ice or uncooked rice. This disorder puts patients at risk of dangerous levels of weight loss, nutritional problems and medical complications, as well as generating high levels of emotional distress.

What now? The end of the honeymoon period

> Our bariatric patients . . .want more; they want more weight loss, more happiness, more ability to eat, more of everything. Many patients . . . have told me that if they were to lose just [some weight], they would want nothing more. Then when they reach [that weight] most want more. They are only human.
>
> Cowan 1998[1]

Many patients experience the first year or so after surgery as a time of great excitement. They feel buoyed up on a wave of optimism and happiness that makes them feel they can take on the world. Their confidence and motivation are unbounded and they revel in the attention of others. The weight is falling off and they are feeling healthier and full of energy. Unfortunately, for most, this honeymoon period comes to an end around 18 months or two years after surgery. By this time, weight loss may have slowed or stopped and people will no longer be commenting on your transformation (they may barely remember what you looked like before you lost weight). Family and friends begin to take your new eating regime and appearance for granted and the regular compliments and encouragement disappear. You will be having fewer follow-ups with your bariatric team, potentially leaving you feeling alone with your worries. Having been swept along by the process of adjusting to surgery, it is now that old problems in your personal life or emotional well-being can re-emerge. It is at this stage that you are perhaps most vulnerable to encountering problems as you face the reality of life post-surgery.

> [The support from the team] . . . was great for the first 28 months, but I do feel very lost and neglected now and yet now is when I

could use more support than for the year after surgery (when your body kind of works to its own accord).

A, gastric bypass

Pushing for more weight loss

It's important to recognise that the aim of bariatric surgery is not to get you down to a 'normal' weight. It is designed to reduce health problems and improve your quality of life. It will not get you to a size 10 and is likely to leave you still significantly overweight. Unfortunately, a proportion of bariatric patients are not happy with the weight loss they achieve; while the thought of losing 45kg may have sounded fantastic before surgery, the reality of being left 30kg overweight may not be what you had banked on.

So, while most bariatric patients will have good improvements in their health and quality of life, 1 in 10 patients with a BMI between 40 and 49 pre-surgery will remain technically obese. Of a group of extremely overweight patients (with BMI over 50 before surgery) 45 per cent will remain obese at five years post-gastric bypass. By ten years post-surgery, almost 60 per cent of highly obese and 20 per cent of obese patients will have a BMI over 35.[58] If you are only interested in the number on the scales, ignoring the medical and quality of life benefits, you are likely to feel pretty frustrated and disappointed.

Seeking to *push* your weight loss beyond what can reasonably be expected from surgery can lead to a whole set of emotional and physical problems. Even if you have achieved more weight loss that you ever could through diet and exercise alone, you may start to see yourself as a failure. Some people start to restrict their food intake excessively (increasing the risk of nutritional problems and serious complications) or exercising compulsively. Of course the other outcome is that people become demoralised and give up, reverting to unhealthy eating habits.

If you are post-surgery and your weight loss has slowed or stopped, go back to the calculation in Chapter 5 showing the weight loss you can expect with surgery. Have you reached that point? If yes, you may need to accept that further weight loss may not be realistic and focus instead on maintaining your weight through regular activity and a healthy, balanced diet. If you haven't lost as much weight as expected, reflect on your progress; have you been limiting high calorie foods? Are you careful to follow the dietitian's advice? Are you getting active a few times a week? If you feel you have gone off track, go back to your food diary and identify the times when your eating has been problematic. Are there specific triggers for overeating that you can modify or manage? Monitoring and recording your food intake will help you get more in control, but you may also need further support from the bariatric dietitian.

Excess skin

Whether through dieting or weight loss surgery, massive weight loss nearly always results in loose skin. The majority of weight loss surgery patients report some problem with excess skin, mainly on the stomach, arms, breasts and thighs, with some patients developing a skin flap that hangs below the knees, and many find this surplus skin very unpleasant and distressing, resulting in self-consciousness and a reluctance to take part in activities where they need to expose their body. Excess skin can impact on mobility, physical comfort during exercise, personal hygiene, libido and feelings of personal attractiveness. Some patients feel that the loose skin is a *greater* problem than their previous large size; they feel unattractive or disgusting and this can inhibit them from starting new relationships.

> I regularly beat myself up for being ugly and fat and feel I look a lot worse now than I did when I was fat but firm.
>
> A, gastric bypass

> I've lost all this weight and I resemble an 80-year old woman. I thought I'd feel sexier but I felt hideous. I felt more depressed at that point than I did when I was fat. I seriously thought about putting the weight back on.
>
> Sarah, quoted in *Times Magazine*, p30[30]

Despite this, most people appear to expect some loose skin and do not regret having had surgery:[59]

> One consequence was excess baggy skin, but it doesn't trouble me and it was expected to a degree.
>
> C, gastric bypass

For most patients it is not reasonable to expect to get rid of loose skin through exercise or diet, and many people, and particularly younger women, express a wish for cosmetic surgery to get rid of excess skin.[60] In the USA in 2005, almost 70,000 bariatric patients had body contouring surgery, mainly breast reduction or lift, abdominoplasty (removal of the skin around the abdomen), lower body lift, and upper arm and thigh lifts. Body contouring surgery involves the surgical removal of excess skin and unwanted fatty deposits after surgery.[61] As with all surgery, these procedures clearly carry risks, such as infection, poor healing,[62] blood clots and scarring, and more complex surgery may need to be staged over a number of months.

Cosmetic surgery can only take place once weight has been stable for a considerable period of time, after which you may be referred for a cosmetic surgery assessment. Patients who have achieved a BMI below 35, with weight stability and good nutritional status do best with body contouring surgery. The success of body contouring depends on maintaining a stable weight, and it is unrealistic to see it as a way of achieving better weight loss or preventing weight regain.

> When I got down to my smallest, if I had been allowed to have . . . plastic surgery I probably would not have as easily regained because space for the fat would have been removed and my mental state may have been better retained.
>
> A, gastric bypass

There are no national guidelines in the UK about body contouring surgery. A recent survey of UK bariatric surgeons[63] suggests that many surgeons have patients who complain about problems with excess skin, though not all surgeons counsel their patients about this issue before surgery. Most bariatric surgeons believe their patients should be able to access body contouring surgery on the NHS, but it is often difficult to get to see a cosmetic surgeon and there is no clear agreement about the criteria patients would need to meet to be eligible for funding. Your bariatric team should provide information about cosmetic surgery[13] but you should not assume that it will be provided automatically.

What to do if things are going wrong

Not all weight loss surgery patients are happy with the outcome; one in ten gastric band patients is uncertain or would not have surgery if they could make the decision again and almost 10 per cent report that their health is worse than before surgery.[64] It's important to bear in mind that the results reported in big research papers may *underestimate* the number of patients who struggle after surgery, who have problems adjusting to the new way of eating or regain a lot of weight, because these people may simply stop attending follow-up meetings with their bariatric team due to feelings of shame or hopelessness.

The first and most important thing to do if you are encountering difficulties is to contact your bariatric team. They should be able to provide you with the information and support you need to start improving the situation. If you are having medical complications, such as pain or frequent vomiting or if you are not restricted in your food intake you may need to see the surgeon for review. The dietitian can help if your eating has become uncontrolled or you are not losing enough weight. If you are feeling very low in mood, or are experiencing problems with compulsive behaviours, you need to speak to your GP urgently to get some help. Remember, these kinds of problems are unlikely to work out on their own; you need to get support in order to resolve the situation. It is not helpful to suffer alone and ignoring a problem can lead to serious medical or emotional complications. The rule of thumb is: if you're worried, talk to someone about it.

There are, of course, also many things you can do to help yourself. In Chapter 6 we looked at a number of strategies you can employ to look after yourself emotionally and you might want to revisit these. Use practical strategies to combat anxiety and promote a sense of control and hopefulness. Take each day as it comes, setting realistic goals to help you make small, steady changes in the right direction.

Techniques for getting back on track

Monitor progress

If you have lost the habit of recording everything you eat and drink, re-start a food diary. It can be immensely helpful in giving you a sense of control and identifying areas where you are becoming unstuck.

Solve problems

Use the problem-solving technique to tackle the difficulties you are facing (see Chapter 6). Be as clear as possible about what the real problem is, then consider all possible solutions. Rate each solution according to how likely it is to work and how helpful it is. Choose the action that seems to give you the best chance of a good outcome and put it into action. Once you've tried that for a time, review how helpful it's been. If it's worked well, carry on; if not, try the next option on your list and so on.

Get support

Join a weight loss surgery support group. Being able to talk through your experiences with people who have been through the same situation can be very reassuring. Other patients can often provide you with helpful tips on how to manage difficulties and you will feel less alone with your problems. If you are not able to get along to a group, join one of the many online forums – you are likely to find that the situation you're experiencing has also been of concern to others.

Make plans

When people feel unhappy or anxious about their situation, they are less likely to make good decisions, so you may need to take extra care to plan and think through how you are managing the dietary and lifestyle changes. If you don't have a plan you are more vulnerable to the 'to hell with it' effect we talked about in Chapter 8. Reduce the risk of overeating by having meal plans for each day of the week. Be very clear about what you will eat if you are away from home, as it may be difficult to access a suitable meal. Use a list (based on your meal plan) whenever you go food shopping, to ensure that you only buy the food you need and are less tempted by special offers or high fat, high sugar foods. Faced with a celebratory meal or trip to a restaurant, make an agreement with yourself about how you will manage the situation. If necessary check the menu beforehand, and be careful with your alcohol consumption as this reduces your inhibitions and you are more likely to make poor food choices.

Make time

If you are having problems because you're simply not finding time to do what you need to do – be it plan meals, getting some exercise, or going to a support group – you need to think about how you prioritise your time and how you communicate your needs to people around you. When you decided to have weight loss surgery it was (hopefully) because you wanted to feel better physically and emotionally. You presumably felt it was time to do something about your life and made some kind of commitment (to yourself and your bariatric team) that you would do what was necessary to make it work. Of course these commitments can easily get lost among the daily demands on our time and energy, but you need to remind yourself again – you can only look after yourself if you have time and emotional resources left after looking after everyone else. Be clear about what you need and ask for it. Go back to the section on assertiveness in Chapter 6 and practise saying 'no' (or if that's too hard 'not now').

Weight loss surgery is a stressful process and many people struggle with the physical and emotional challenges. It is important to know the potential problems when you embark on surgery as this is an essential component of your informed decision. It is natural that you would hope or expect that 'it won't happen to me', but many people do have physical complications or difficulties adjusting to life after surgery and you need to consider how you would cope if it happened to you. Some patients may wish they'd never gone ahead, but for the majority of weight loss surgery patients the challenges are overcome and the balance of positive and negative outcomes ultimately make it a worthwhile accomplishment.

Carry out a post-surgery MOT

A few months after surgery, think about completing a personal MOT, to review goals and to check whether you are making the progress you want. Spend some time thinking about the statements below to help identify any problems or vulnerable areas. Catching any difficulties early will give you a better chance of getting on top of them.

Rate each of the statements on the scale below and circle the number that best represents your experience:

Key: **SD – strongly disagree; D – disagree; NS – not sure; A – agree; SA – strongly agree**

		SD	D	NS	A	SA
1.	I feel confident about managing my eating.	1	2	3	4	5
2.	I am able to exercise regularly.	1	2	3	4	5
3.	I feel miserable now I can't eat.	5	4	3	2	1
4.	I have had good support from my friends.	1	2	3	4	5
5.	My partner brings home treats for me, like chocolate and ice cream.	5	4	3	2	1
6.	I am not able to do any physical activity.	5	4	3	2	1
7.	I am losing weight steadily.	1	2	3	4	5
8.	I have more energy and feel better in myself.	1	2	3	4	5
9.	I still feel self-conscious and anxious about going out.	5	4	3	2	1
10.	It feels like my friends are jealous of the way I look.	5	4	3	2	1
11.	I try to walk or do some exercise most days.	1	2	3	4	5
12.	I worry I'm drinking too much alcohol.	5	4	3	2	1
13.	I am able to plan and organise my meals.	1	2	3	4	5
14.	I feel tearful and hopeless about the future.	5	4	3	2	1
15.	My partner and/or friends have expressed concern about how I eat.	5	4	3	2	1
16.	I have felt alone in coping with surgery.	5	4	3	2	1
17.	I am very happy with the outcome of surgery.	1	2	3	4	5

		SD	D	NS	A	SA
18.	I am gaining weight.	5	4	3	2	1
19.	I love all the attention and compliments I'm getting.	1	2	3	4	5
20.	My health has improved.	1	2	3	4	5
21.	I feel I have lost the pleasure in my life.	5	4	3	2	1
22.	It's been hard, but worth it.	1	2	3	4	5
23.	I sometimes lose control of my eating.	5	4	3	2	1
24.	I am feeling positive and optimistic.	1	2	3	4	5
25.	My partner has been supportive all the way.	1	2	3	4	5
26.	I am experiencing problematic complications.	5	4	3	2	1
27.	My overall health has deteriorated.	5	4	3	2	1
28.	I feel more confident socially.	1	2	3	4	5
29.	I find it hard to motivate myself to exercise.	5	4	3	2	1
30.	I feel uncomfortable with the way other people react to me now.	5	4	3	2	1

Scoring

Overall satisfaction and weight loss: add up your scores from statements 7, 17, 18, 22 and 26.

A high score indicates that you feel generally positive with the outcome of surgery. You are losing weight and coping well with the changes to diet and lifestyle. A low score suggests that you have not had a good outcome so far. Perhaps you are not losing weight as well as you hoped, are experiencing medical complications or day-to-day symptoms such as vomiting or discomfort. Try talking to other weight loss surgery patients and get support from your bariatric team.

Eating behaviour: add up your scores from statements 1, 13, 15 and 23.

A high score suggests that you feel confident about managing your diet well and are not experiencing major problems in adjusting to your new relationship with food. A low score suggests that you are struggling to cope with the changes to your eating and may be having problems with snacking or loss of control of your eating. This puts you at risk of poor weight loss and medical complications. It's important that you concentrate on getting your eating back on track. Start a food diary and speak to your bariatric dietitian.

Emotional well-being: add up your scores from statements 3, 9, 12, 14, 21 and 24.

A high score suggests that you are feeling positive and happy. You are not experiencing difficult emotional reactions to the changes in lifestyle or the experience of weight loss. A low score suggests that you are struggling with the emotional impact of surgery, possibly due to the emotional strain of the restricted diet or as the result of emotional or social consequences of weight loss. You may be using alcohol to cope with distress. A low score indicates that you may be suffering from depression or anxiety and it's vitally important that you speak to your GP about how you're feeling.

Health: add up your scores from statements 8, 20 and 27.

A high score suggest that you have experienced an improvement in your health and are feeling more energetic and active. A low score suggests that your health has got worse or stayed the same and this may be preventing you from engaging in physical activity. Speak to your GP or bariatric team about getting additional support.

Social well-being: add up your scores from statements 10, 19, 28 and 30.

A high score suggests that you are feeling more socially confident and comfortable in your social activities. A low score suggests that you have experienced some negative reactions from people around you since surgery or are feeling uncomfortable with people's response to your weight loss. This may simply mean you are still adjusting to your new image or may be a sign of more deep-seated difficulties relating to your experience of your body or close relationships. If you feel that family or friends are reacting unhelpfully, you may need to be more assertive about your needs; some relationships take a little time to adjust. If the problem is raising painful feelings or memories and you are also scoring low on the emotional well-being questions, you should speak to your GP about accessing psychological support.

Physical activity: add up your scores from statements 2, 6, 11 and 29.

A high score suggests that you have been able to establish a good exercise routine and are able to engage in some physical activity regularly.

You are feeling motivated and recognise the importance of regular exercise. A low score suggests that for physical, social or emotional reasons you are struggling to engage in regular physical activity. You may still be feeling self-conscious or low mood may be affecting your motivation or confidence. Exercise is an important component to the changes needed to make surgery successful so it's important to get some support. Going for a walk each day is a realistic and effective way of building up motivation and fitness. You can also speak to your GP about whether you can access help in establishing an exercise routine.

Support from others: add up your scores from statements 4, 5, 16 and 25.

A high score suggests that friends and family have supported your efforts and that you have not felt alone with the challenges your face. Continue to be open and assertive about your need for support. A low score suggests that you perhaps do not have people to support you or that people have not always been helpful. You may be feeling alone in coping with the challenges you face. People may have tried to encourage you to eat the wrong kinds of foods or reacted negatively to changes in your lifestyle. Either way it's essential that you get support and encouragement from others. Joining a support group and talking to your bariatric team can help you feel less alone. If your partner is responding very unhelpfully to the post-surgery changes, it may be useful to seek relationship counselling. The contact details for Relate counselling service are in Chapter 11.

If you're are having problems in any of the areas considered above, it's important to remember it's very unlikely that you will be the first person to have gone through it. Often simply talking to someone about the difficulties you're encountering will help you feel less anxious and a little more able to cope. Many of these problems will not resolve themselves without help, but with assistance from your bariatric team, GP, support group and friends they can be overcome. You may have access to a support group through your bariatric service and patient organisations, such as BOSPA and WLSInfo, also run support groups – you can find your nearest group on their websites. Don't allow feelings of embarrassment, shame or hopelessness prevent you from seeking the help you need.

11

Taking control: FAQs and resources

Throughout this book, you have been encouraged to consider each aspect of weight loss surgery with all its benefits and pitfalls. It is certainly true that surgery is not right for everyone and I hope you now have the information you need to assess whether you are a good candidate. For some the weight loss produced by surgery allows improvements in health and emotional well-being that are life-changing; for others the results are disappointing or even devastating. Unlike any other kind of surgery, the outcome is almost entirely down to your ability to establish lifelong changes in your relationship with food and approach to exercise. The physical aspect of weight loss surgery provides a tool to support these changes, but does not produce these transformations simply through the surgeon's efforts. To put it another way, the surgery won't magically give you control over your eating, but it may allow you to take control. In this way, your hopes and expectations, commitment, motivation, emotional resilience and support network will determine your success with surgery more definitively than the surgeon's skills. This chapter covers frequently asked questions about weight loss surgery and information about useful sources of support to aid you on your journey.

Frequently asked questions

What would my doctor want me to know about weight loss surgery?

The bottom line is that your surgeon and bariatric team want you to know that weight loss surgery is not a magic cure, it works only if you make it work! It's challenging and requires permanent changes to the way you deal with food. It's not a cure to all the problems in your life, but it can be a very effective way of producing sustainable weight loss and reducing weight-related illnesses. The surgery involved (depending on the procedure) can carry potentially life-threatening risks; you can only reasonably accept these risks for the medical benefits, not for cosmetic reasons. Weight loss surgery will not get you down to a perfect size 10 and you may be left considerably overweight.

All bariatric procedures have been shown to result in good improvements in weight-related health problems and are associated with greater life expectancy. Patients also report feeling more energetic and with less bodily pain, all contributing to a better quality of life. Remember that, in general, improvements in health after surgery are dependent on weight loss and you may not get a good outcome if you don't comply with the dietary guidelines or if you have poor weight loss. There is more information about the health benefits in Chapter 9.

How do I find a bariatric surgeon?

This will depend on whether you plan to have surgery privately or through the NHS, though in either case the first conversation should be with your GP who can check whether you meet the NICE criteria and discuss your options. If you have NHS funding you may be offered a choice of possible surgical centres around your area. You may want to consider waiting times, location, your experience of different hospitals and the size of the service when making a decision. If you are going private you need to be very clear about what is included in the surgery package; does it cover multidisciplinary assessment; pre-surgery investigations; a flexible number of fills (if you are having a gastric band); dietetic support and access to a support group?

Whichever bariatric service you go to, you may want to ask about the number of surgeries they carry out each year. Research shows that the lowest rates of complications are associated with bariatric centres that deal with high numbers of patients (over 100) each year. High risk patients, including those with a very high BMI, older patients and patients with heart or respiratory problems should have surgery at a high volume specialist centre. See Chapter 4 for more information.

What is the best procedure for me?

Deciding on the best bariatric procedure will depend on a number of factors and many people find that their preference changes as they go through the assessment process. You will need to balance the risks and benefits with each procedure; in general the gastric bypass and biliopancreatic diversion/duodenal switch (BPD/DS) offer the best weight loss and health benefits, but also carry the highest risk, while the gastric band is reversible and has lower risks, but offers less in terms of weight loss and health improvements. The sleeve gastrectomy sits between the other two procedures in terms of risks and benefits. Some people want the rapid weight loss offered by the gastric bypass, while others may feel steadier weight loss with the band will give them time to adjust to their new body image. The choice of procedure will also be influenced by your health problems and any history of abdominal surgery. Your eating habits will also affect the decision; for example, if you eat a lot of chocolate, crisps and high fat foods, the gastric band may not give you a good outcome. See Chapter 7 for detailed information about the different bariatric procedures.

How much weight will I lose with surgery?

Many bariatric patients overestimate surgical weight loss and unrealistically high expectations can leave you frustrated and demoralised and vulnerable to depression, problematic eating and weight regain. Overall surgery offers average weight loss of around 60 per cent excess weight; somewhat more with gastric bypass or BPD/DS and somewhat less with the sleeve gastrectomy and gastric band. Excess weight is worked out as the difference between your pre-surgery weight and the weight that would give you a BMI of 25. So weight loss surgery does not get you down to a 'normal' weight and you may still be significantly overweight. If you have a pre-surgery BMI over 50 and achieve the expected weight loss, you are still likely to have a BMI over 35 (that is, you will remain technically obese). It is expected that patients will regain some weight in the longer term, so by ten years after surgery, average *maintained* weight loss is between 14 and 25 per cent total pre-surgery weight, but this compares to a weight *gain* of 2 per cent body weight in patients receiving standard care for obesity in the same time scale. Check your realistic weight loss goal in Chapter 5.

Will I have to go on a diet before surgery?

There are two reasons why you may be asked to change your eating habits before surgery. First, a number of bariatric services expect you to demonstrate your motivation and commitment by losing some weight during the assessment process. This is generally combined with advice to follow a healthy, balanced diet, having three regular meals and cutting out snacks, sugary drinks and takeaways. As well as showing the team that you are able to lose weight, it also helps prepare you for the post-surgery changes to your diet.

Second, most surgeons expect you to follow a special pre-surgery diet for one or two weeks before surgery. This diet is designed to shrink the size of your liver by reducing its stores of glycogen and water. The surgeon has to move the liver to access the stomach during weight loss surgery, so by reducing the size of the liver you reduce the risk of surgical complications. The details of the pre-surgery diet depend on your bariatric team, but it will be low in carbohydrates, sugar and fat. Some services recommend a 'milk only' diet, while others offer a range of diet options (see Chapter 7 for more information). The dietitian will give you detailed information about what you can and can't eat at this stage. It's very important that you stick to the diet conscientiously; just one large meal will undo the good work.

Will I be able to eat normally after surgery?

In order to be successful with weight loss surgery you will need to make dramatic changes to the way you eat and your relationship with food. Immediately after surgery you will be on a liquid diet, only slowly incorporating thicker liquids, pureed and soft foods over the following weeks and months before moving on to a more regular varied diet. This gives your stomach pouch time to heal or the band to settle. Eating solid foods or overeating during these early stages can reduce the effectiveness of surgery or cause serious complications. You need to have regular meals, eating slowly and thoughtfully, chewing food carefully and avoiding drinking during meals. Serving yourself overly large portions can mean you gradually train your new stomach to accept more food. A poor diet can lead to loss of muscle mass, hair loss and dry skin.

After a couple of months the bariatric team will expect you to establish a healthy balanced diet, incorporating a wide variety of foods such as lean protein (such as fish, meat and eggs and low fat dairy), a range of vegetables, salad and carbohydrates and only small amounts of fats and sugars. Including protein in every meal helps to prevent the loss of lean muscle mass and enhances feelings of fullness. This is the foundation for your new eating habits, so it's important to base your diet around healthy nutritious foods, rather than slipping back to old habits of relying on high calorie foods, which may feel easier to digest or more comforting.

The restriction on food intake created by surgery will give you strong feedback on what and how much you can eat. Feelings of hunger are weakened and satiety signals are clearer. You should feel full on much smaller amounts of food and less hungry between meals. Some people find it hard to tolerate foods like bread, rice, pasta and meat. A degree of trial and error in what works for you is normal, but you need to avoid repeatedly 'testing the boundaries' of the surgical restriction. Relying on soft, sweet foods may feel easier but will mean that you do not achieve such good weight loss.

The basics are reasonably simple; have three meals daily, eat a variety of foods, choose whole foods, avoid convenience and processed food as much as possible, and don't have high calorie drinks, but as well as the physical effect of restricted food intake, you will also need to adjust to the emotional impact of the loss of food as comfort and pleasure. The psychological consequences of having food removed as a source of release and comfort may be particularly difficult if you have a history of emotional or binge eating. See Chapters 8 and 10 for information about changes to your approach to food after surgery.

Will I still enjoy food?

Inevitably your relationship with food will change after weight loss surgery. You will need to work hard to ensure that you have regular nutritious meals and that you eat food slowly and thoughtfully. Many patients feel less hungry, more in control of their eating and less vulnerable to binge episodes. Before surgery prospective bariatric patients often speak of wanting to eat to live rather than live to eat, and for many weight loss surgery offers this. There is also evidence that gastric bypass in particular decreases *hedonic hunger,* the *wanting* hunger rather than the *needing* or physical hunger.

The potential downside of these changes is that some people get very low in mood in response to loss of pleasure from food or seek to find pleasure or relief from stress in other unhelpful behaviours, such as excessive consumption of alcohol or drugs, compulsive shopping or sexual activity. As some people put it, food is no longer your friend – you cannot turn to it for comfort when you are feeling low or alone.

Is it normal to vomit after eating?

Frequent vomiting is not considered an inevitable part of life after weight loss surgery and can lead to problems such as band slippage, nutritional problems, damage to the oesophagus and tooth decay. Vomiting is usually due to eating or drinking too quickly or too much, or choosing foods that cannot be easily chewed down too soon after surgery. If you experienced continued and frequent vomiting you need to get advice from your bariatric team.

What is dumping syndrome?

Dumping syndrome occurs after gastric bypass surgery when people eat sugary foods. It causes nausea, vomiting, palpitations, weakness, sweating, stomach cramps, faintness and diarrhoea. Dumping occurs in around 50–70 per cent of gastric bypass patients. The experience of dumping can be very unpleasant and may leave you feeling washed out and exhausted for a number of hours, but, on the up side, it quickly trains people not to consume sugary, high calorie foods.

You can reduce the problem of dumping by eating more protein, limiting sugary foods like chocolate, cake, ice cream and biscuits; including wholegrain foods in your diet; avoiding sugary drinks; and having small regular meals. It also helps to eat slowly and avoid drinking for 20 minutes after your meal.

Is it still possible to overeat after surgery?

Weight loss surgery is not a magical solution to uncontrolled eating. While surgery should definitely restrict how much you can eat at one time, a surprisingly high proportion of bariatric patients report that they continue to snack or use drinks to wash down food so they can eat more. Others eat less but still consume a lot of high fat or high sugar foods. These behaviours are common in patients whose weight loss plateaus early or who show excessive weight regain.

Patients who have a history of binge eating or who use food to cope with difficult emotions are most at risk of experiencing loss of control over their eating after surgery. Though you are unable to consume the very large amounts of food that would constitute a binge episode before surgery, nevertheless some people continue to eat to the point of feeling uncomfortably full or fall into a pattern of snacking through the day. Frequent grazing, relying on surgery to provide 'enough' restriction, continued emotional eating, and testing boundaries or 'cheating' the restrictions rather than taking personal responsibility for your choices, will mean that you don't achieve the best weight loss.

I've been told I have a binge eating disorder, what is this?

A binge episode is characterised by the consumption of an excessive amount of food in a relatively short period of time with the individual experiencing a loss of control over their eating, followed by feelings of shame or guilt. If binge episodes occur frequently (at least twice a week) and cause distress, the person is said to have a *binge eating disorder*. Binge eating disorder is associated with emotional difficulties and body image distress.

It is thought that between 20 and 30 per cent of weight loss surgery candidates have a binge eating disorder. Some people diagnosed with binge eating disorder before surgery continue to experience some loss of control of their eating after surgery or fall into a pattern of grazing through the day and this has been associated with poorer weight loss and higher risk of weight regain.

People who have suffered with bulimia (when binge episodes are followed by attempts to compensate for the excessive calories consumed during the binge, by vomiting, laxative use or excessive exercise) are expected to have been clear of these behaviours for at least 12 months before surgery. For more information about binge eating and other forms of disordered eating see Chapter 5.

Why do I need to take vitamin supplements?

Nutritional problems are not as much of an issue with the gastric bypass as originally thought, but there is a risk of nutritional difficulties with all procedures, and most particularly with the malabsorptive procedures. You will need to take daily supplements including a good quality multi-vitamin together with B^{12}, calcium, folic acid, zinc and iron for the rest of your life and maintain a nutritious, balanced diet that is high in protein.

Nutritional deficiencies are more likely to occur if you are vomiting frequently or if you are not able to take in enough food and are losing weight rapidly, and can lead to hair loss, fatigue, loss of muscle mass, headaches, palpitations and depression. In rare cases vitamin B^1 deficiency, associated with too rapid weight loss, frequent vomiting and excessive alcohol consumption, can result in permanent brain damage.

Where can I get recipe ideas?

There are a number of cookery books written especially for weight loss surgery patients available online. There are also various websites that offer ideas and advice, such as ☝ www.bariatriccookery.com. Always check that the recipes and suggestions are consistent with advice from your bariatric dietitian.

Can my teenage daughter have weight loss surgery?

Extremely overweight children and adolescents are at risk of major health problems and emotional and social difficulties. Adolescents may be offered weight loss surgery if they have a high BMI and serious health problems; have reached the final stages of puberty; are near or at their adult height; are able to understand the implications and risks of surgery; are highly motivated to make changes; and have good support from their family. However, there is little information about the potential long-term impact on teenagers' emotional health, metabolic function and nutritional status, so surgery is only considered if all attempts at mainstream treatment, including intensive support with dietary and behaviour change and increased physical activity, have been unsuccessful. See Chapter 4 for more information.

Children who are overweight, from pre-schoolers to teenagers, can get help and support from MEND. MEND stands for 'Mind, Exercise, Nutrition ... Do it!' and they run healthy lifestyle programmes for children and families in local communities. They can be contacted on ☎ 0800 230 0263 or ☝ www.mendcentral.org.

What should I do if my partner is against me having surgery?

It's important that you have encouragement and support from the people around you after weight loss surgery, so having a partner who is set against it could raise a lot of difficulties and make it harder for you to make successful changes.

There seem to be three main reasons why partners reject the idea of surgery. First, he or she may just feel very concerned about the risks of surgery. In this case it is often helpful for them to attend hospital appointments and a support group with you to get a clearer idea of what's involved. Reliable information about the risks of surgery and how the risks balance against the health benefits of weight loss is often all that's needed to get them on side. Encourage them to read through Chapters 7, 9 and 10.

Second, your partner may be worried about your ability to cope with surgery. Sometimes those close to us know our strengths and weaknesses better than we do ourselves. Has your partner expressed concern about the need to change your eating habits or the emotional impact of surgery? If so, are their concerns justified? Do you also have some worries about whether you will be able to stick to the post-surgery diet? Do you fear that the loss of food could mean a loss of pleasure in your life?

Finally, some partners object to the idea of surgery because they fear it will impact on the relationship. He or she may feel threatened by the prospect of you losing weight and becoming more attractive to others, worried that it will destabilise the relationship. Others don't like the idea of their partner taking control and making decisions for themselves. There's a risk that insecure or controlling partners will consciously or otherwise sabotage your best efforts and threaten the success of surgery, particularly if they have a history of reacting negatively to previous diet attempts.

The important thing is that you and your partner continue to talk openly and honestly about surgery. Your partner may have reasonable and realistic worries about you going ahead with surgery, even if you're confident it's the best decision. If you can't resolve the issue by talking to your partner and doing some research together, it may be helpful to talk it through with the support of a counsellor. You can organise relationship counselling through Relate (⌂ www.relate.org.uk ☎ 0300 100 1234).

Will I be left with excess skin when I lose weight?

Whether through dieting or weight loss surgery, massive weight loss nearly always results in loose skin. The majority of weight loss surgery patients report some problem with excess skin, mainly on the stomach, arms, breasts and thighs. Some people find this surplus skin very unpleasant and distressing. Excess skin can affect mobility, physical comfort, personal hygiene, libido and feelings of personal attractiveness.

Some patients will want to think about cosmetic surgery to deal with the excess skin. Body contouring surgery involves the surgical removal of excess skin and unwanted fatty deposits. As with all surgery, these procedures carry risks, including infection, poor healing, blood clots and scarring.

Patients who achieve a stable weight below BMI 35 and good nutritional status do best with body contouring surgery. The success of body contouring depends on maintaining a stable weight and it is unrealistic to see it as a way of achieving better weight loss or preventing weight regain. At the current time there are no national guidelines for body contouring in the UK. Your bariatric team should provide information about cosmetic surgery, but you should not assume that it will be provided automatically on the NHS.

Will weight loss surgery affect the medication I take?

You may need to make changes to any diabetes medication around the time of surgery and you will be given advice about how to manage this. Malabsorptive surgery, including gastric bypass and BPD/DS can affect the absorption of certain medications, including certain psychiatric and anti-epilepsy medications, and your bariatric team will talk to you and other involved health professionals about how to adjust for this. You may need to take your medication in liquid or soluble form.

Will I be able to have children after surgery?

You need to avoid getting pregnant for two years after surgery as there could be nutritional difficulties for you and your baby. You must take precautions against pregnancy even if you've previously been told that you can't get pregnant, as weight loss surgery can make you more fertile. Most studies conclude that pregnancy after weight loss surgery is safe for both the mother and baby with lower rates of gestational diabetes and pre-eclampsia. However, gastric bypass patients will need to take particular care with their nutritional supplements to prevent the baby having a neural tube defect. See Chapter 9 for more information.

The bariatric team has recommended that I have psychological therapy before surgery, why is this?

If you have become aware of a tendency to eat in response to difficult emotions, if you use food to comfort or calm yourself, or you have binge episodes where you lose control of your eating, you may be vulnerable to continued problematic eating and so it would be helpful to tackle these behaviours before going ahead with weight loss surgery. You may need psychological therapy or counselling (ideally with the support of a therapist specialised in disordered eating) to deal with these problem behaviours and learn more helpful ways of coping with stress and upset.

If you suffer from depression or anxiety you should not assume that this will be resolved by surgery. While many patients report feeling less distressed and anxious, bariatric surgery is not a treatment for emotional difficulties. It is suggested that where depression or other emotional problems are primarily due to the impact of obesity on self-esteem, quality of life, relationships and so on, then it is likely to resolve following surgery. Where the emotional difficulties are unrelated to the weight issue and/or began before onset of the weight problem, they are less likely to improve spontaneously after surgery. Being significantly depressed will reduce the emotional resources you can access to cope with the demands of surgery and you need to be in the best possible emotional state before you proceed. Think about speaking to your GP about referral to local psychological therapy services and look at the techniques for managing stress and upset in Chapter 6.

How can I find a psychologist or counsellor?

If you want to start psychological therapy before or after weight loss surgery, your GP is always the first point of call. He/she can discuss the issues concerning you and if necessary make a referral to an NHS service. Some GP surgeries have a counsellor or psychologist working within the practice. Alternatively your doctor could register you with the 'Beating the Blues' online CBT course for depression and anxiety (www.beatingtheblues.co.uk).

If you plan to see someone privately, you might need to do some research into the kind of therapy you'd find helpful. Cognitive-behavioural therapy (CBT) has evidence for its effectiveness in treating anxiety, depression and eating problems. CBT tends to focus on the problems you face 'here and now' and is often relatively short term. If you want therapy to give you space to reflect on the impact of early life experiences on your emotional well-being and behaviour patterns, you might look at longer-term psychotherapy.

You will need to ensure that the person you are seeing is properly qualified and there are a number of organisations that regulate and monitor the training of counsellors, clinical psychologists and psychotherapists. The British Psychological Society (BPS) website allows you to search for chartered clinical psychologists in your area (⌨ www.bps.org.uk). Clinical psychologists should also be registered with the Health Professions Council (HPC ✎ www.hpc-uk.org). The equivalent organisation representing psychotherapists and counsellors in the UK is the British Association for Counselling and Psychotherapy (BACP ✎ www.bacp.co.uk). The British Association for Behavioural & Cognitive Psychotherapies (BABCP) provides information about CBT and helps you find an accredited cognitivebehavioural therapist (✎ www.babcp.com).

Why have I been refused weight loss surgery?

There are a number of reasons why the bariatric team may feel that you're not suitable for surgery at this time. This may be related to your eating habits; poor motivation; reluctance to take responsibility for making the necessary changes to your diet; or poor understanding of the demands of surgery. Severe mental health problems, such as schizophrenia or bipolar disorder; current drug or alcohol dependency; or a history of self-harm may mean that you are less able to tolerate and comply with the post-surgical restrictions. People with dementia or a significant learning disability are likely to struggle with understanding and maintaining a suitable healthy diet. You can be confident that the bariatric team will carry out a thorough assessment of your needs and will make a decision based on your best interests.

I don't really want surgery, should I give dieting another go?

It is important that you don't go ahead with surgery if you're not ready for it and maybe you want to give dieting one last chance. Depending on your BMI, weight loss of around 10 per cent of initial body weight can offer good health benefits, but you need to be aware that it will take time and effort. The best weight management approaches combine exercise, diet and behavioural strategies,[1] focusing on realistic and sustainable lifestyle changes for weight loss of ½ –1kg a week.

Though you won't get the same degree of weight loss as with surgery, you can still achieve sufficient weight loss to show improvements in your health.[2] Even weight loss of 10 per cent body weight can produce clinically significant improvements in diabetic control, blood lipids,[3,4] blood pressure[5] and lung function,[6] as well as reducing the risk of developing type 2 diabetes[7] and cancer[8,9] and improving health-related quality of life.[10] However if you have a high BMI you may find that traditional weight management approaches are less effective[11] and you may realistically need to lose more than 10 per cent body weight to get sustained health benefits.[12]

Speak to your GP about the support available to you. If you believe you have binge eating disorder (see Chapter 5), you need to get this managed before you can achieve success with any form of weight management treatment. Some areas offer specialist weight management services and these may offer better outcomes compared with people receiving less support, but research evidence suggests that most people regain the weight over time.[13] A weight management programme including behavioural intervention, dietary advice, exercise and skills for preventing relapse will typically produce weight loss of around ½kg a week during the programme and 60–70 per cent of this weight loss is maintained for the first year.[14] However, follow up over the next three to five years tends to show weight regain to original levels[15] and *weight cycling* may exacerbate problems with eating control.[16]

If you're embarking on another diet, spend some time thinking about blocks to weight loss in the past. These may include[17] being dissatisfied with (realistic) levels of weight loss; difficulty managing food cravings; eating in response to stress or upset; binge eating; not using problem-solving skills; low confidence in being able to control eating; and feeling that the effort to lose weight is greater than the benefits of weight loss. These blocks are less about what diet you start and much more to do with your expectations and confidence. As we've seen, losing weight and maintaining weight loss over time is challenging and many of the skills and strategies we've talked about through this book will be equally relevant for dieters. Make sure you have realistic expectations and bear the following principles in mind:

- Don't start a diet that involves cutting out whole foods groups, carbohydrates, fat and so on. In fact, don't go on a *diet* at all; all diets come to an end and you may feel hopeless about succeeding before you even start, especially if you have a long history of diet attempts. What you are looking for are sensible, moderate changes to your eating that over the months and years will allow you to lose weight slowly and steadily and that fit in with your lifestyle. Most of the commercial slimming clubs now focus on a flexible, healthy approach to losing weight and many people find the weekly support helpful.
- Don't set weight goals, set goals for lifestyle change. Focus on improvements in your quality of life, confidence or fitness rather than on your weight.
- Recognise that weight loss is going to be slow. It's very tempting to want quick results, but restricting your food intake too much will make it much more difficult to sustain the changes over time and if you break your diet the weight is likely to ping right back on.
- Your weight loss will slow down or stop at some point and this is a frequent break point with diets. If you view this as a natural part of the process you will not become so demoralised; persevere with the changes to your diet and increase your activity levels if possible.

- Avoid rigid food rules, such as 'I will never eat chocolate/pizza/cake', as this makes you crave these foods and increases the risk of overeating when you break the rule.
- Weigh yourself regularly, to monitor your progress and to reduce the risk of weight regain[12] but not so often that you get upset about normal variations in weight – once a week should be fine.
- Use the stress management skills and problem solving techniques in Chapter 6 to deal with upsets and problems.
- Find yourself a buddy to support and encourage you. Slimming clubs can help you feel less alone in your efforts.
- Keep a food diary (see Chapter 5) to monitor your efforts and keep you on track.
- Think long term and keep your goals in mind. In the context of the rest of your life, there is no value in beating yourself up over a slip in your diet. The more you tell yourself that you can't do it, the less emotional strength you'll have to keep the changes going.

For most people the challenge is not in losing the weight but in *maintaining* weight loss. Unfortunately, research evidence suggests that the majority of people regain the lost weight within five years. You can help keep the weight off by maintaining positive lifestyle changes, including regular physical activity and low levels of sedentary time, sticking with a low fat diet, recording your food and drink intake and weighing yourself regularly.

What is a gastric pacemaker?

The gastric pacemaker consists of a device, inserted into the stomach via keyhole surgery, which delivers a series of small electrical impulses to the stomach. These impulses produce neurohormonal changes that increase feelings of fullness. The idea is that it teaches people to be satisfied with smaller portions. It is a new procedure and currently is only available in a few private hospitals. The device also sends information about food intake and physical activity to a computer to support long-term changes in behaviour. The advantages of the system are that it is reversible, carries fewer surgical risks and provides direct feedback about eating behaviour and exercise. As yet there is little evidence on long-term effectiveness or potential problems.

Is cosmetic surgery an alternative to weight loss surgery?

Cosmetic surgeries, such as tummy tucks and liposuction, are not effective in producing sustainable weight loss and are not used as treatment for obesity.[18] With liposuction, for example, the percentage of body fat, total fat mass, stomach and thigh circumference and skin folds are all significantly reduced six weeks after surgery, but there is already a reduced effect by six months, and by one year there is no difference between the liposuction group and no-treatment group. Fat does tend to stay off the hips and thighs for longer but this fat is redistributed to the stomach.[19]

How can I find a support group?

Many bariatric services have their own support group and you should be able to get information about this from the team. Patient organisations also run support groups that you are welcome to attend before and after surgery. These include BOSPA (⌁ www.bospa.org) and WLSInfo (⌁ www.wlsinfo.org.uk); you can find details of support groups in your area on their websites.

A–Z of useful organisations and websites

Al-Anon ⌁ www.al-anonuk.org.uk ☏ 020 7403 0888. Supports people whose lives are affected by other people's drinking.

Alcoholics Anonymous (AA) ⌁ www.alcoholics-anonymous.org.uk ☏ 0845 769 7555. Offers support to people who have an alcohol abuse problem.

Be Mindful ⌁ www.bemindful.co.uk. Useful source of mindfulness resources and information about local courses.

British Association for Behavioural & Cognitive Psychotherapies (BABCP) ⌁ www.babcp.com. Provides information about CBT and helps you find an accredited cognitive-behavioural therapist in your area.

British Association for Counselling and Psychotherapy (BACP) ⌁www.bacp.co.uk ☏ 01455 883316. Represents psychotherapists and counsellors in the UK.

British Obesity Surgery Patients Association (BOSPA) ⌁ www.bospa.org. Information and support for bariatric patients, pre- and post-surgery.

British Psychological Society (BPS) ⌁ www.bps.org.uk ☏ 0116 2549568. The BPS represents psychologists in the UK. The website allows you to search for chartered clinical and counselling psychologists in your area.

BuddyPower ⌁ www.buddypower.net. Online resource and forum for people trying to manage their weight, including weight loss surgery patients.

Compassionate Mind Foundation ⌁ www.compassionatemind.co.uk. Mainly aimed at therapists but has links to a range of helpful websites.

Dr Foster ⌁ www.drfosterhealth.co.uk. Provides information about hospitals, consultants and social care services to help people make informed choices.

Get Self Help ⌁ www.get.gg. A range of CBT self-help resources, including an online CBT self-help course, downloadable relaxation/mediation resources and information about disordered eating.

Health Professions Council (HPC) ⌁ www.hpc-uk.org. Registers health professionals including psychologists and dietitians.

MEND ⌁ www.mendcentral.org ☏ 0800 230 0263. Runs healthy lifestyle programmes for children and families in local communities.

Men's Advice Line ⌁ www.mensadviceline.org.uk ☎ 0808 8010327. Supports men affected by domestic violence.

Mind ⌁ www.mind.org.uk ☎ 0845 766 0163. Provides information, support and advice to people with mental health problems and can guide you towards local services.

Mindfulness-based Cognitive Therapy ⌁www.mbct.co.uk. Provides mindfulness resources and information about mindfulness-based cognitive therapy.

Narcotics Anonymous (UK) ⌁ www.ukna.org ☎ 0300 999 1212. Provides support for people who have a drug problem and addicts in recovery.

NHS Choices ⌁ www.nhs.uk/conditions/obesity. This website includes information about the causes and consequences of obesity. There is comprehensive information about weight loss surgery (www.nhs.uk/Conditions/weight-loss-surgery) and an easy-to-use BMI calculator (www.nhs.uk/tools/pages/healthyweightcalculator). Also see www.nhs.uk/livewell for information about healthy eating and exercise.

Refuge ⌁ www.refuge.org.uk ☎ 0808 2000 247. Supports women and children affected by domestic violence.

Relate ⌁ www.relate.org.uk ☎ 0300 100 1234. Provides relationship counselling, family therapy and sex therapy.

Samaritans ⌁ www.samaritans.org ☎ 08457 90 90 90. Provides emotional support to people in distress 24 hours a day.

Self-compassion ⌁ www.self-compassion.org. Website run by leading practitioner in self-compassion, Dr Kristin Neff, offering resources and guidance.

Weight Concern ⌁ www.weightconcern.com. A good source of information about overweight, obesity and maintaining a healthy lifestyle.

Weight Loss Surgery Information and Support (WLSInfo) ⌁ www.wlsinfo.org.uk. Information and support for bariatric patients pre- and post-surgery.

Further reading

1. The obesity epidemic and weight loss surgery

1. World Health Organisation (2011) *Obesity and overweight. Fact sheet N° 311*. Available at http://www.who.int/mediacentre/factsheets/fs311/en.
2. Cheltenham Science Festival (2007) Dating the obesity epidemic. Accessed at http://www.telegraph.co.uk/science/science-news/3296662/When-DID-we-start-getting-fat.html.
3. The Information Centre for Health and Social Care (2011) Statistics on obesity, physical activity and diet: England, 2011. Available at http://data.gov.uk/dataset/statistics-on-obesity-physical-activity-and-diet-england-2011.
4. Foresight Report (2007) *Tackling obesities. Future Choices Project*. Accessed at www.bis.gov.uk/foresight/our-work/projects/published-projects/tackling-obesities.
5. National Obesity Observatory (2010) *The economic burden of obesity*. Available at www.noo.org.uk.
6. DeJong W (1980) The stigma of obesity: the consequences of naïve assumptions concerning the causes of physical deviances. *Journal of Health and Social Behaviour* 21:75–87.
7. Puhl R and Brownell KD (2001) Bias, discrimination and obesity. *Obesity Research* 9:788–805.
8. Welbourn R, Fiennes A, Kinsman R and Walton P (2011) *The United Kingdom National Bariatric Surgery Registry. First Registry Report to March 2010*. Henley on Thames: Dentrite Clinical Systems.
9. Puhl RM and Heuer CA (2011) Public opinion about laws to prevent weight discrimination in the United States. *Obesity* 19(1):74–82.
10. Crandell CS and Moriarty D (1995) Physical illness stigma and social rejection. *British Journal of Social Psychology* 34:67–83.
11. Sikorski C, Luppa M, Glaesmer H *et al.* (2011) The stigma of obesity in the general public and its implications for public health – a systematic review. *BMC Public Health* 11:661.
12. National Institute for Health and Clinical Excellence (2007) Commissioning guide. Implementing NICE guidance. Bariatric surgical service for the

treatment of people with severe obesity. Available at www.nice.org.uk/usingguidance/commissioningguides/bariatric/assumptions.jsp.

13. Christou NV, Sampalis JS, Liberman M *et al.* (2004) Surgery decreases long-term mortality, morbidity, and health care use in morbidly obese patients. *Annals of Surgery* 240:416–423.

14. Narbro K, Agren G, Jonsson E *et al.* (1999) Sick leave and disability pension before and after treatment for obesity: A report from the Swedish Obese Subjects (SOS) study. *International Journal of Obesity and Related Metabolic Disorders* 23:619–624.

15. Brownell KD and Wadden TA (1992) Etiology and treatment of obesity: understanding a serious, prevalent and refractory disorder. *Journal of Consulting and Clinical Psychology* 60:435–442.

16. Torgerson JS and Sjostrom L (2001) The Swedish Obese Subjects (SOS) study – rationale and results. *International Journal of Obesity* 25(1):S2–54.

17. Karlsson J, Taft C, Ryden A *et al.* (2007) Ten-year trends in health-related quality of life after surgical and conventional treatment for severe obesity: the SOS intervention study. *International Journal of Obesity and Related Metabolic Disorders* 31(8):1248–1261.

18. Adams KF, Schatzkin A, Harris TB *et al.* (2006) Overweight, obesity, and mortality in a large prospective cohort of persons 50 to 71 years old. *New England Journal of Medicine* 355:763–778.

19. Volger S, Vetter ML, Dougherty M *et al.* (2011) Patients' preferred terms for describing their excess weight: discussing obesity in clinical practice. *Obesity* doi:10.1038/oby.2011.217.

20. Carlson NR (2007) Ingestive behaviour. In *Physiology of Behaviour* 9th edn. Needham Heights, MA: Allyn & Bacon.

21. Ochner CN, Gibson C, Shanik M *et al.* (2010) Changes in neurohormonal gut peptides following bariatric surgery. *International Journal of Obesity* 1–14.

22. Schweitzer DH, Dubois EF, van den Doel-Tanis N and Oei HI (2007) Successful weight loss surgery improves eating control and energy metabolism: a review of the evidence. *Obesity Surgery* 17:533–539.

23. Noel PH and Pugh JS (2002) Management of overweight and obese adults. *British Medical Journal* 325:757–761.

24. Wilding J (1997) Science, medicine and the future: obesity treatment. *British Medical Journal* 315:997–1000.

2. Obesity: a normal response to an abnormal situation?

1. Swinburn BA, Sacks G, Hall KD *et al.* (2011) The global obesity epidemic: shaped by global drivers and local environments. *Lancet* 378:804–814.

2. Wansink B, Painter JE and North J (2005) Bottomless bowls: why visual cues of portion size may influence intake. *Obesity Research* 13(1):93–100.

3. Epstein LH, Truesdale R, Wojcik A *et al.* (2003) Effect of deprivation on hedonistic and reinforcing value of food. *Physiology and Behaviour* 78:221–227.

4. Centers for Disease Control and Prevention (2004) Trends in the intake of energy and macronutrients – United States. *Morbidity and Mortality Weekly Report* 53:80–82.

5. Wansink B and Chandon P (2006) Can low-fat nutrition labels lead to obesity? *Journal of Marketing Research* 43(4):605–617.

6. Fowler SP, Halada GV and Fernandes G (2011) Aspartame consumption is associated with elevated fasting glucose in diabetes-prone mice. Abstract No. 0788-P. American Diabetes Association 71st Scientific Sessions, June 2011, San Diego, California.

7. Fowler SP, Williams K and Hazuda HP (2011) Diet soft drink consumption is associated with increased waist circumference in the San Antonio Longitudinal Study of Aging. Available at http://ww2.aievolution.com/ada 1101/index.cfm?do=abs.viewAbs&abs=10061. American Diabetes Association 71st Scientific Sessions, June 24–28, 2011, San Diego, California.

8. House of Commons Health Committee – Third Report in Session 2003–4.

9. Ogden J, Stavrinaki M and Stubbs J (2009) Understanding the role of life events in weight loss and weight gain. *Psychology, Health & Medicine* 14(2):239–249.

10. The NS and Gordon-Larsen P (2009) Entry into romantic partnership is associated with obesity. *Obesity (Silver Spring)* 17(7):1441–1447.

11. Brown WJ, Hockey R and Dobson AJ (2010) Effects of having a baby on weight gain. *American Journal of Preventative Medicine* 38(2):163–170.

12. Yanovski JA, Yanovski SZ, Sovik KN *et al.* (2000) A prospective study of holiday weight gain. *New England Journal of Medicine* 342:861–867.

13. Tremblay MS, Warburton DER, Janssen I *et al.* (2011) New Canadian physical activity guidelines. *Applied Physiology, Nutrition and Metabolism* 36:36–46.

14. The NHS Information Centre (2011) *Statistics on obesity, physical activity and diet: England 2011*. Available at www.ic.nhs.uk/webfiles/publications/ 003_Health_Lifestyles/opad11/Statistics_on_Obesity_Physical_Activity_ and_Diet_England_2011_revised_Aug11.pdf.

15. Williamson DF, Madans J, Anda RF *et al.* (1991) Smoking cessation and severity of weight gain in a national cohort. *New England Journal of Medicine* 324:739–745.

16. Audrain-McGovern J and Benowitz NL (2011) Cigarette smoking, nicotine, and body weight. *Clinical Pharmacology & Therapeutics* 90(1):164–168.

17. Lee Moffitt Cancer Centre and Research Institute (2000) *Forever Free. Booklet 3: A guide to remaining smoke free*. Available at http://www. smokefree.gov/pubs/ffree3.pdf.

18. Kruger J, Blank H and Gillespie C (2006) Dietary and physical activity behaviours among adults successful at weight loss maintenance. *International Journal of Behaviour Nutrition & Physical Activity* 3(1):17.

19. Rutter H (2011) Where next for obesity? *The Lancet* 378:746–747.

20. Kennedy GC (1972) The regulation of food intake. *Advances in Psychosomatic Medicine* 7:91–99.

21. Sumithran P, Prendergast LA, Delbridge E *et al.* (2011). Long-term persistence of hormonal adaptations to weight loss. *New England Journal of Medicine* 365(17): 1597–1604.

22. Ogden J (2003) *The psychology of eating: from healthy to disordered behaviour*. Oxford: Blackwell.

23. Shade ED, Ulrich CM, Wood B *et al.* (2004) Frequent intentional weight loss is associated with lower natural killer cell cytotoxicity in postmenopausal

women: possible long-term immune effects. *Journal of the American Dietetic Association* 104(6):903–912.

24. Adam T and Epel E (2007) Stress, eating and the reward system. *Physiology and Behaviour* 91:449–458.

25. Schur E, Heckbert S and Goldberg J (2010) The association of restrained eating with weight change over time in a community-based sample of twins. *Obesity (Silver Spring)* 18(6):1146–1152.

26. Greeno CG and Wing RR (1994) Stress-induced eating. *Psychological Bulletin* 115:444–464.

27. Stambor Z (2006) Stressed out nation. *Monitor on Psychology* 37: 28–29.

28. Kandiah J, Yake M, Jones J and Mayer M (2006) Stress influences appetite and comfort food preference in college women. *Nutritional Research* 26(3):118-123.

29. Wardle J, Chida Y, Gibson EL *et al.* (2011) Stress and adiposity: a meta-analysis of longitudinal studies. *Obesity* 19(4): 771–778.

30. Stice E, Presnell K, Shaw H and Rohde P (2005) Psychological and behavioural risk factors for obesity onset in adolescent girls: a prospective study. *Journal of Consulting and Clinical Psychology* 73:195–202.

31. Hepworth R, Mogg K, Brignell C and Bradley B (2010) Negative mood increases selective attention to food cue and subjective appetite. *Appetite* 54:134–142.

32. Dallman MF, Pecoraro NC and la Fleur SE (2005) Chronic stress and comfort foods: self-medication and abdominal obesity. *Brain Behaviour and Immunity* 19:275–280.

33. Rowland NE and Antelman SM (1976) Stress-induced hyperphagia and obesity in rats: a possible model for understanding human obesity. *Science* 191:310–312.

34. Stone AA and Brownell KD (1994) The stress-eating paradox: multiple daily measurements in adult males and females. *Psychological Health* 9:425–436.

35. Brown G (2000) *The Energy of Life*. London: Flamingo.

36. Epel E, Jimenez S, Brownell K *et al.* (2004) Are stress eaters at risk for the metabolic syndrome? *Annals of the New York Academy of Science* 1032:208–210.

37. Gluck ME (2006) Stress response and binge eating disorder. *Appetite* 46:26–30.

38. Felitti VJ, Anda RF, Nordenberg D *et al.* (1998) Relationship of childhood abuse and household dysfunction to many of the leading causes of death in adults. The Adverse Childhood Experiences (ACE) study. *American Journal of Preventative Medicine* 14(4):245–258.

39. Williamson DF, Thompson TJ, Anda RF *et al.* (2002) Body weight and obesity in adults and self-reported abuse in childhood. *International Journal of Obesity and Related Metabolic Disorders* 26(8):1075–1082.

40. Rich-Edwards JW, Spiegelman D, Lividoti-Hibert EN *et al.* (2010) Abuse in childhood and adolescence as a predictor of type 2 diabetes in adult women. *American Journal of Preventative Medicine* 39(6):529–536.

41. Lee JM, Gebremariam A, Keirns CC *et al.* (2010) Getting heavier, younger: trajectories of obesity over the life course. *International Journal of Obesity* 34:614–623.

42. Harrington JW, Nguyen VQ, Paulson JF et al. (2010) Identifying the 'tipping point' age for overweight pediatric patients. *Clinic Pediatrics (Philadelphia)* 49(7):638–643.

43. Craigie AM, Lake AA, Kelly SA et al. (2011) Tracking of obesity-related behaviours from childhood to adulthood: a systematic review. *Maturitas* 70(3):266–284.

44. Freedman DS, Khan LK, Dietz WH et al. (2001) Relation of childhood obesity to coronary heart disease risk factors in adulthood: the Bogalusa Heart Study. *Pediatrics* 108(3):712–718.

45. The Information Centre for Health and Social Care (2011) Statistics on obesity, physical activity and diet: England, 2011. Available at http://data. gov.uk/dataset/statistics-on-obesity-physical-activity-and-diet-england-2011.

46. Griffiths LJ and Hawkins SS (2009) Using the Millennium Cohort Study to examine growth and obesity across childhood. *Kohort: CLS Cohort Studies Newsletter*. Institute of Education, University of London.

47. Cook S, Weitzman M, Auinger P et al. (2004) Prevalence of the metabolic syndrome phenotype in adolescents: findings from the third National Health and Nutrition Examination Survey. *Archives of Pediatric and Adolescent Medicine* 157:821–827.

48. Must A, Jacques PF, Dallal GE et al. (1992) Long-term morbidity and mortality of overweight adolescents: a follow-up of the Harvard Growth Study of 1922 to 1935. *New England Journal of Medicine* 327:795–797.

49. National Obesity Observatory (2011) *Obesity and mental health*. Available to download at www.noo.org.uk.

50. Van Wijnen LGC, Boluijt PR, Hoeven-Mulder HB et al. (2010) Weight status, psychological health, suicidal thoughts, and suicide attempts in Dutch adolescents: results from the 2003 E-MOVO Project. *Obesity* 18(5):1059–1061.

51. Burke MA, Heiland FW and Nadler CM (2010) From 'overweight' to 'about right': evidence of a generational shift in body weight norms. *Obesity* 18(6):1226–1234.

52. Christakis NA and Fowler JH (2007) The spread of obesity in a large social network over 22 years. *New England Journal of Medicine* 357:370–379.

53. Maximova K, McGrath JJ, Barnett T et al. (2008) Do you see what I see? Weight status misperception and exposure to obesity among children and adolescents. *International Journal of Obesity* 32:1008–1015.

54. Hayden-Wade HA, Stein RI, Ghaderi A et al. (2005) Prevalence, character-istics and correlates of teasing experiences among overweight children vs. non-overweight peers. *Obesity Research* 13:1381–1392.

55. Althuizen E, Mireille M, van Poppel N et al. (2009) Correlates of absolute and excessive weight gain during pregnancy. *Journal of Women's Health* 18(10):1559–1566.

56. Siega-Riz AM, Viswanathan M, Moos MK et al. (2009) A systematic review of outcomes of maternal weight gain according to the institute of medicine rec-ommendations: birthweight, fetal growth, and postpartum weight retention. *American Journal of Obstetrics and Gynecology* 201(4):339.e1–339.e14.

57. Simkin-Silverman LR, Wing RR, Boraz MA and Kuller LH (2003) Lifestyle intervention can prevent weight gain during menopause: results from a

5-year randomized clinical trial. *Annals of Behavioural Medicine* 26(3): 212–220.

58. US Department of Health and Human Services Office of Women's Health. *Polycystic ovary syndrome (PCOS) factsheet.* Available at www.womenshealth. gov/publications/our-publications/fact-sheet/polycystic-ovary-syndrome.

59. Ali ZA and Radebold K (2009) Insulinoma. Accessed on 28.11.2011 at http:// emedicine.medscape.com.article/283039-overview.

60. Ruetsch O, Viala A, Bardou H *et al.* (2005) Psychotropic drugs induced weight gain: a review of the literature concerning epidemiological data, mechanisms and management. *Encephale* 31(4):507–516.

61. Farooqi IS and O' Rahilly S (2007) Genetic factors in human obesity. *Obesity Reviews* 8(1):37–40.

62. Walley AJ, Asher JE and Froguel P (2009) The genetic contribution to non-syndromic human obesity. *Nature Reviews Genetics* 10:431–442.

63. Montague CT, Farooqi JS, Whitehead JP *et al.* (1997) Congenital leptin deficiency is associated with severe early-onset obesity in humans. *Nature* 387:903–908.

64. Vaisse C, Clement K, Guy-Grand B and Froguel P (1998) A frameshift mutation in human MC4R is associated with a dominant form of obesity. *Nature Genetics* 20:113–114.

65. Branson R, Potoczna N, Kral JG *et al.* (2003) Binge eating as a major phenotype of melanocortin 4 receptor gene mutations. *New England Journal of Medicine* 348(12):1096–1103.

66. Frayling TM, Timpson NJ, Weedon MN *et al.* (2007) A common variant in the FTO gene is associated with body mass index and predisposes to childhood and adult obesity. *Science* 316 (5826):889–894

67. Geller F, Reichwald K, Dempfle A *et al.* (2004) Melanocortin-4 receptor gene variant l103 is negatively associated with obesity. *American Journal of Human Genetics* 74(3):572–581.

68. Mizuta E, Kokubo Y, Yamanaka I *et al.* (2008) Leptin gene and receptor gene polymorphisms are associated with sweet preference and obesity. *Hypertension Research* 31:1069–1077.

69. González JE (2011) Genes and obesity: a cause and effect relationship. *Endocrinological Nutrition* 5(9):492–496.

3. 'I just want a normal life': the impact of obesity

1. Sturm R (2002) The effects of obesity, smoking, and problem drinking on chronic medical problems and health care costs. *Health Affairs* 21(2): 245–253.

2. Sturm R and Wells KB (2001) Does obesity contribute as much to morbidity as poverty or smoking? *Public Health* 115:229–295.

3. Welbourn R, Fiennes A, Kinsman R and Walton P (2011) *The United Kingdom National Bariatric Surgery Registry. First Registry Report to March 2010.* Henley on Thames: Dentrite Clinical Systems.

4. National Institute for Health and Clinical Excellence (2006) *Obesity: guidance on the prevention, identification, assessment and management of overweight and obesity in adults and children.* Available at www.nice.org. uk/nicemedia/live/11000/30365/30365.pdf

5. The Hormone Foundation ◌www.hormone.org/diabetes.

6. American Heart Association ◌www.americanheart.org.

7. British Heart Foundation ◌www.bhf.org.uk.

8. The Information Centre for Health and Social Care (2010) *NHS statistics on obesity, physical activity and diet: England, 2010.* Available at www.ic.nhs.uk/webfiles/publications/opad10/Statistics_on_Obesity_Physical_Activity_and_Diet_England_2010.pdf.

9. Grundy SM, James I, Cleeman JI, Daniels SR *et al.* (2005) Diagnosis and management of the metabolic syndrome: an American Heart Association/ National Heart, Lung and Blood Institute scientific statement. *Circulation* 112:2735–2752.

10. Ford ES, Giles WH and Dietz WH (2002) Prevalence of the metabolic syndrome among US adults: findings from the third National Health and Nutrition Examination Survey. *Journal of the American Medical Association* 287(3):356–359.

11. Sareli AE, Cantor CR, Williams NN *et al.* (2011) Obstructive sleep apnea in patients undergoing bariatric surgery – a tertiary centre experience. *Obesity Surgery* 21(3):316–327.

12. Vortmann M and Eisner MD (2008) BMI and health status among adults with asthma. *Obesity* 16:146–152.

13. Jiang L, Rong J, Wang Y *et al.* (2011) The relationship between body mass index and hip osteoarthritis: a systematic review and meta-analysis. *Joint Bone Spine* 79(2):150–155.

14. Peltonen M, Lindroos AK and Torgenseon (2003) Musculoskeletal pain in the obese: a comparison with the general population and long-term changes after conventional and surgical obesity treatment. *Pain* 104: 549–557.

15. Lakdawalla DN, Bhattacharya J and Goldman DP (2004) Are the young becoming more disabled? *Health Affairs* 23(1):168–176.

16. Cancer Research UK. Information and statistics on the link between obesity and cancer can be found at http://info.cancerresearchuk.org/ healthyliving/obesityandweight/howdoweknow/.

17. Adams LA and Angulo P (2006) Treatment of non-alcoholic fatty liver disease. *Postgraduate Medicine Journal* 82(967): 315–22.

18. Pournaras DJ, Manning L, Bidgood K *et al.* (2010) Polycystic ovary syndrome is common in patients undergoing bariatric surgery in a British centre. *Fertility and Sterility* 94(2):e41.

19. O'Dwyer V, Farah N, Fattah C *et al.* (2011) The risk of caesarean section in obese women analyses by parity. *European Journal of Obstetrics Gynaecology and Reproductive Medicine* 158(1):28–32.

20. Catalano PM (2007) Management of obesity in pregnancy. *Obstetrics and Gynaecology* 109:419–433.

21. National Obesity Observatory (2010) Maternal obesity and maternal health. Available at www.noo.org.uk/NOO_about_obesity/maternal_obesity/ maternalhealth.

22. Dwyer PL, Lee ETC and Hay DM (1988) Obesity and urinary incontinence in women. *BJOG: An International Journal of Obstetrics and Gynaecology* 95:91–96.

23. Cummings JM and Rodning CB (2000) Urinary stress incontinence among obese women: review of pathophysiology therapy. *International Urogynecology Journal and Pelvic Floor Dysfunction* 11:41–44.
24. Zaninotto P, Wardle H, Stomamatakis E *et al.* (2006) Forecasting obesity to 2010. www.erpho.org.uk/download/public/15199/1/forecastingobesityto 2010.pdf.
25. Abdullah A, Wolfe R, Stoelwinder JU *et al.* (2011) The number of years lived with obesity and the risk of all-cause and cause-specific mortality. *International Journal of Epidemiology* doi: 10.1093/ije/dyr018.
26. Fontaine KR, Redden DT, Wang C *et al.* (2003) Years of life lost due to obesity. *Journal of the American Medical Association* 289(2):187–193.
27. Fabricatore AN, Wadden TA, Sarwer DB *et al.* (2005) Health-related quality of life and symptoms of depression in extremely obese persons seeking bariatric surgery. *Obesity Surgery* 15:304–309.
28. Petry NM, Barry D, Pietrzak RH and Wagner JS (2008) Overweight and obesity are associated with psychiatric disorders: results from the national epidemiologic survey on alcohol and related conditions. *Psychosomatic Medicine* 70:288–297.
29. Kalarchian MA, Marcus MD, Levine MD *et al.* (2007) Psychiatric disorders among bariatric surgery candidates: relationship to obesity and functional health status. *American Journal of Psychiatry* 164:328–334.
30. Dong C, Li W-D, Li D *et al.* (2006) Extreme obesity is associated with attempted suicides: results from a family study. *International Journal of Obesity* 30:388–390.
31. National Obesity Observatory (2011) *Obesity and mental health.* Available to download at www.noo.org.uk.
32. Stunkard A and Mendelson M (1967) Obesity and the body image: characteristics of disturbances in the body image of some obese people. *American Journal of Psychiatry* 123:1296–1300.
33. Sarwer DB, Thompson JK and Cash TF (2005) Body image and obesity in adulthood. *Psychiatric Clinics of North America* 28:69–87.
34. Davidson KK, Schmaltz DL, Young LM and Birch LL (2008) Overweight girls who internalise fat stereotypes report low psychological well-being. *Obesity* 16(2):30–38.
35. Stunkard AJ and Sorensen TIA (1993) Obesity and socioeconomic status – a complex relation. *New England Journal of Medicine* 329:1036–1037.
36. Rand CS and MacGregor AM (1991) Successful weight loss following obesity surgery and the perceived liability of morbid obesity. *International Journal of Obesity* 15:577–579.
37. Puhl RM and Brownell KD (2001) Bias, discrimination and obesity. *Obesity Research* 9:788–805.
38. Puhl RM and Latner JD (2007) Stigma, obesity and the health of the nation's children *Psychological Bulletin* 133:557–580.
39. Gortmaker SL, Must A, Perrin JM *et al.* (1993) Social and economic consequences of overweight in adolescence and young adulthood. *New England Journal of Medicine* 329(14):1008–1012.
40. Baum CL and Ford WF (2004) The wage effects of obesity: a longitudinal study. *Health Economics* 13:885–899.

41. Sarlio-Lahteenkorva S and Lahelma E (1999) The association of body mass index with social and economic disadvantage in women and men. *International Journal of Obesity* 28:445–449.
42. Jones E, Farina A, Haslorf A *et al.* (1984) *Social stigma: the psychology of marked relationships.* New York: Freeman.
43. Crandell CS and Moriarty D (1995) Physical illness stigma and social rejection. *British Journal of Social Psychology* 34:67–83.
44. http://yaleruddcenter.org/resources/upload/docs/what/reports/Rudd_Policy_Brief_Weight_Bias.pdf
45. Phelan JC, Link BG and Dovidio JF (2008) Stigma and prejudice: one animal or two? *Social Science and Medicine* 67:358–367.
46. Puhl RM and Heuer CA (2010) Obesity stigma: important considerations for public health. *American Journal of Public Health* 100:1019–1028.
47. Vartanian LR and Novak SA (2011) Internalised societal attitudes moderate the impact of weight stigma on avoidance of exercise. *Obesity* 19(4):757–762.
48. Haines J, Neumark-Sztainer D, Eisenberg ME and Hannan PJ (2006) Weight teasing and disordered eating behaviour in adolescents: longitudinal findings from Project EAT (Eating Among Teens). *Pediatrics* 117:209–215.
49. Chen EY, Bocchieri-Ricciardi LE, Munoz D *et al.* (2007) Depressed mood in class III obesity predicted by weight-related stigma. *Obesity Surgery* 17(5):669–671.

4. Accessing weight loss surgery

1. National Institute for Health and Clinical Excellence (2006) *CG43 Obesity: Guidance on the prevention, identification, assessment and management of overweight and obesity in adults and children. Quick reference guide 2 for the NHS.* Available at www.nice.org.uk. Patient information relating to this guidance *Information about NICE clinical guideline 43: treatment for people who are overweight* can be accessed at www.nice.org.uk/nicemedia/pdf/CG43publicinfo1.pdf.
2. Nguyen NT, Paya M, Stevens CM *et al.* (2004) The relationship between hospital volume and outcome in bariatric surgery at academic medical centers. *Annals of Surgery* 240(4):586–594.
3. National Institute for Health and Clinical Excellence (2007) *Bariatric surgical service for the treatment of people with severe obesity. Commissioning guide implementing NICE guidance.* At www.nice.org.uk/media/87F/65/BariatricSurgery.
4. Welbourn R, Fiennes A, Kinsman R and Walton P (2011) *The United Kingdom National Bariatric Surgery Registry. First Registry Report to March 2010.* Henley on Thames: Dentrite Clinical Systems.
5. Must A and Strauss R (1999) Risks and consequences of childhood and adolescent obesity. *Journal of Obesity and Related Metabolic Disorders* 23:S2–11.
6. Baker JL, Olsen LW and Sorensen TL (2007) Childhood body-mass index and the risk of coronary heart disease in adulthood. *New England Journal of Medicine* 357(23):2329–2337.

7. Kim RJ, Langer JM, Baker AW *et al.* (2008) Psychosocial status in adolescents undergoing bariatric surgery. *Obesity Surgery* 18:27:33.
8. Inge TH, Krebs NF, Garcia VF *et al.* (2004) Bariatric surgery for severely overweight adolescents: concerns and recommendations. *Pediatrics* 114:217–223.
9. Woolford SJ, Clark SJ, Gebremariam A *et al.* (2010) To cut or not to cut: physicians' perspectives on referring adolescents for bariatric surgery. *Obesity Surgery* 20:937–942.
10. Baur LA and Fitzgerald DA (2010) Recommendations for bariatric surgery in adolescents in Australia and New Zealand. *Journal of Paediatrics and Child Health* 46:704–707.
11. Aikenhead A, Lobstein T and Knai C (2011) Review of current guidelines on adolescent bariatric surgery. *Clinical Obesity* 1:3–11.
12. Prochaska JO and DiClemente CC (1992) *Stages of change in the modification of problem behaviors.* Newbury Park, CA: Sage.

5. Assessment for weight loss surgery

1. National Institute for Health and Clinical Excellence (2006) *CG43 Obesity: Guidance on the prevention, identification, assessment and management of overweight and obesity in adults and children. Quick reference guide 2 for the NHS*. Available at www.nice.org.uk.
2. Jones-Corneille LR, Wadden TA, Sarwer DB *et al.* (2010) Axis I psychopathology in bariatric surgery candidates with and without binge eating disorder: Results of a structured clinical interview. *Obesity Surgery* DOI 10.1007/s11695-010-0322-9.
3. Sarwer DB, Wadden TA, Fabricatore AF (2005) Psychosocial and behavioural aspects of bariatric surgery. *Obesity Research* 13:639–648.
4. Kalarchian MA, Courcoulas A, Levine M *et al.* (2007) Presurgery psychiatric disorders are associated with smaller reductions in BMI at six months after gastric bypass. *Surgery for Obesity and Related Diseases* 3:280.
5. Rosik CH (2005) Psychiatric symptoms among prospective bariatric surgery patients: rates of prevalence and their relation to social desirability, pursuit of surgery and follow-up attendance. *Obesity Surgery* 15:677–683.
6. Herpertz S, Kielmann R, Wolf AM *et al.* (2003) Does obesity surgery improve psychosocial functioning? *International Journal of Obesity* 27:1300–1314.
7. Shiri S, Gurevich T, Feintuch U and Beglaibter N (2007) Positive psychological impact of bariatric surgery. *Obesity Surgery* 17:663–668
8. Herpertz S, Kielmann R, Wolf AM *et al.* (2004) Do psychosocial variables predict weight loss or mental health after obesity surgery? A systematic review. *Obesity Research* 12:1554–1569.
9. Adams TD, Gress RE, Smith SC *et al.* (2007) Long-term mortality after gastric bypass surgery. *New England Journal of Medicine* 357(8):753–761.
10. Stevens T, Spavin S, Scholtz S and McClennan L (2012) Your patient and weight-loss surgery. *Advances in Psychiatric Treatment* 18:418–425.
11. Hagedorn JC, Encarnacion B, Brat GA *et al.* (2007) Does gastric bypass alter alcohol metabolism? *Surgery for Obesity and Related Diseases* 3:543–548.

12. Norris L (2007) Psychiatric issues in bariatric surgery. *Psychiatric Clinics of North America* 30:717–738.
13. Allison KC, Wadden TA, Sarwer DB *et al.* (2006) Night eating syndrome and binge eating disorder among persons seeking bariatric surgery: prevalence and related features. *Surgery for Obesity and Related Diseases* 2(2):153–158.
14. Saunders R, Johnson L and Teschner A (1998) Prevalence of eating disorders among bariatric surgery patients. *Eating Disorders* 6:309–317.
15. Wadden TA, Faulconbridge LF, Jones-Corneille LR *et al.* (2011) Binge eating disorder and the outcome of bariatric surgery at one year: a prospective, observational study. *Obesity* 19:1220–1228.
16. Colles SL, Dixon JB and O'Brien PE (2008) Grazing and loss of control related to eating: two high-risk factors following bariatric surgery. *Obesity* 16(3):615–622.
17. Kalarchian MA, Wilson GT, Brolin RE *et al.* (2000) Assessment of eating disorders in bariatric surgery candidates: self-report versus interview. *International Journal of Eating Disorders* 28:465–469.
18. Van Hout GCM, Boekestein P, Fortuin FAM *et al.* (2006) Psychosocial functioning following bariatric surgery. *Obesity Surgery* 16:787–794.
19. White MA, Kalarchian MA, Masheb RM *et al.* (2010) Loss of control over eating predicts outcomes in bariatric surgery patients: a prospective, 24-month follow-up study. *Journal of Clinical Psychiatry* 71:175–184.
20. Kalarchian MA, Marcus MD, Wilson GT *et al.* (2002) Binge eating among gastric bypass patients at long-term follow-up. *Obesity Surgery* 12:270–275.
21. Allison KC, Lundgren JD, O'Reardon JP *et al.* (2010) Proposed diagnostic criteria for night eating syndrome. *International Journal of Eating Disorders* 43(3):241–247.
22. Stunkard AJ and Allison KC (2003) Two forms of disordered eating in obesity: binge eating and night eating. *International Journal of Obesity and Related Metabolic Disorders* 27:1–12.
23. Lundgren JD, Allison KC, Crow S *et al.* (2006) Prevalence of the night eating syndrome in a psychiatric population. *The American Journal of Psychiatry* 163:156–158.
24. Rand CSW, MacGregor AMC and Stunkard AJ (1997) The night eating syndrome in the general population and among prospective obesity surgery patients. *International Journal of Eating Disorders* 22:65–69.
25. Walfish S (2004) Self-assessed emotional factors contributing to increased weight gain in pre-surgical bariatric patients. *Obesity Surgery* 14:1402–1405.
26. Sogg S and Mori DL (2008) Revising the Boston Interview: incorporating new knowledge and experience. *Surgery for Obesity and Related Diseases* 4:455–463.
27. Scholtz S, Bidlake L, Morgan J *et al.* (2007) Long-term outcomes following laparoscopic adjustable gastric banding: preoperative psychological sequelae predict outcome at five-year follow-up. *Obesity Surgery* 17(9):1220–1225.
28. Wadden TA and Sarwer DB (2006) Behavioural assessments of candidates for bariatric surgery: a patient-oriented approach. *Obesity (Silver Spring)* 14(2):S53–62.

29. Macias JA, Vaz Leal FJ, Lopez-Ibor JJ *et al.* (2004) Marital status in morbidly obese patients after bariatric surgery. *German Journal of Psychiatry* 7(3):22–27.
30. Sabbioni MEE, Dickson MH, Eychmuller S *et al.* (2002) Immediate results of health related quality of life after vertical banded gastroplasty. *International Journal of Obesity* 26:277–280.
31. Rand CS, Kowalske K and Kuldau JM (1984) Characteristics of marital improvement following obesity surgery. *Psychosomatics* 25:221–226.
32. Bauchowitz AU, Gonder-Frederick LA, Olbrisch M-E *et al.* (2005) Psychosocial evaluation of bariatric surgery candidates: a survey of present practices. *Psychosomatic Medicine* 67:825–832.
33. Karmali S, Kadikoy H, Brandt ML and Sherman V (2011) What is my goal? Expected weight loss and comorbidity outcomes among bariatric surgery patients. *Obesity Surgery* 21:595–603.
34. Buchwald H, Avidor Y, Braunwald E *et al.* (2004) Bariatric surgery: a systematic review and meta-analysis. *Journal of the American Medical Association* 292(14):1724–1737.
35. Suter M, Calmes J-M, Paroc A *et al.* (2009) Results of Roux-en-Y gastric bypass in morbidly obese vs superobese patients. *Archives of Surgery* 144(4):312–318.
36. Sjöström L, Lindroos A-K, Peltonen M *et al.* (2004) Lifestyle, diabetes and cardiovascular risk factors 10 years after bariatric surgery. *New England Journal of Medicine* 351(26):2683–2693.
37. Wansink B and Cheney MM (2005) Super bowls: serving bowl size and food consumption. *Journal of the American Medical Association* 293(14):1727–1728.
38. Wansink B and van Ittersum K (2008) The perils of plate size: waist, waste, and wallet. Available at http://www.smallplatemovement.org/doc/big_bowls.doc.
39. Tudor-Locke C and Bassett DR (2004) How many steps/day are enough? Preliminary pedometer indices for public health. *Sports Medicine* 34(1):1–8.
40. Cooper Z, Fairburn CG and Hawker DM (2004) *Cognitive-behavioural treatment of obesity: a clinician's guide.* London: Guilford Press.
41. Odom J, Zalesin KC, Washington TL *et al.* (2010) Behavioral predictors of weight regain after bariatric surgery. *Obesity Surgery* 20:349–356.

6. Looking after your emotional well-being

1. The section on compassionate mind training is based on the work of Paul Gilbert and his colleagues. See Gilbert P (2009) *The compassionate mind.* London: Constable & Robinson. A detailed handout outlining the principles of compassionate mind training, *Training our minds in, with and for compassion: an introduction to concepts and compassion-focussed exercises* (Paul Gilbert and colleagues, 2010). Accessed at www.compassionatemind.co.uk/resources.
2. Wise RA (2006) Role of brain dopamine in food reward and reinforcement. *Philosophical Transactions of the Royal Society Biological Sciences* 361:1149–1158.

3. Hyman SE, Malenka RC and Nestler EJ (2006) Neural mechanisms of addiction: the role of reward-related learning and memory. *Annual Review of Neuroscience* 29:565–598.
4. Depue RA and Morrone-Strupinsky JV (2005) A neurobehavioural model of affiliative bonding. *Behavioural & Brain Sciences* 28:313–395. Cited in Gilbert.[1]
5. Kabat-Zinn J (1990) *Full catastrophe living: using the wisdom of your body and mind to face stress, pain and ill*ness. New York: Delta.
6. Linehan MM (1993) *Dialectical behavior therapy*. New York: Guilford Press.
   Hayes SC (2004) *Get out of your head and into your life: the new acceptance and commitment therapy*. New York: New Harbinger.
   Segal Z, Williams M and Teasdale J (2002) *Mindfulness-based cognitive therapy for depression*. London: Guilford Press.
7. Williams M, Teasdale J, Segal Z and Kabat-Zinn J (2007) *The mindful way through depression: freeing yourself from chronic unhappiness*. New York: Guilford Press.
8. Generally attributed, possibly inaccurately, to Dr Seuss.
9. Gurung R (2006) *Health psychology: a cultural approach*. Belmont, CA: Thomson Wadsworth.
10. Gilbert P and Proctor S (2006) Compassionate mind training for people with high shame and self-criticism: overview and pilot study of a group therapy approach. *Clinical Psychology and Psychotherapy* 13: 353–379.
11. Dryden W and Constantinou D (2004) *Assertiveness set by step*. London: Sheldon Press.
12. Blumenthal JA, Michael A, Babyak A *et al.* (2007) Exercise and pharmacology in the treatment of major depressive disorder. *Psychosomatic Medicine* 69:587–596.
    Dunn AL, Trivedi MH and O'Neal HA (2001) Physical activity dose-response effects of depression and anxiety. *Medicine and Science in Sports and Exercise* 33(6):587–597.
13. Strohle A (2009) Physical activity, exercise, depression and anxiety disorders. *Journal of Neural Transmission* 116:777–784.
14. Johnson W and Krueger R (2007) The psychological benefits of vigorous exercise: a study of discordant MZ twin pairs. *Twin Research and Human Genetics* 10(2):1832–4274.
15. Craig R, Mindell J and Hirani V (2008) *Health survey of England: physical activity and fitness*. The NHS Information Centre.
16. Gill A and Safranek S (2010) Clinical inquires: does exercise alleviate symptoms of depression? *Journal of Family Practice* 59(5):530–531.
17. Rendi M, Szabo A, Szabo T *et al.* (2008) Acute psychological benefits of aerobic exercise: a field study into the effects of exercise characteristics. *Psychology, Health & Medicine* 13(2):180–184.
18. Lazarus RS and Folkman S (1984) *Stress, appraisal and coping*. New York: Springer.
19. Neely ME, Schallert DL, Mohammed SS *et al.* (2009) Self-kindness when facing stress: the role of self-compassion, goal regulation and support in college students well-being. *Motivation and Emotion* 33:88–97.

20. Ciarrochi JV and Bailey A (2008) *A CBT practitioner's guide to ACT: how to bridge the gap between cognitive behavioral therapy and acceptance and commitment therapy*. Oakland, CA: New Harbinger Publications.
21. Li X, Wei L and Soman D (2010) Sealing the emotions genie: the effects of physical enclosure on psychological closure. *Psychological Science* 21(8): 1047–1050.
22. Seligman MEP (2003) *Authentic happiness: using the new positive psychology to realize your potential for lasting fulfilment*. London: Nicholas Brealey Publishing. Further information about positive psychology can be found at www.authentichappiness.org.
23. Emmons RA and McCullough ME (2003) Counting blessings versus burdens: experimental studies of gratitude and subjective well-being in daily life. *Journal of Personality and Social Psychology* 84:377–389.
24. Vgontzas AN, Duanping L, Pejovic S *et al.* (2009) Insomnia with objective short sleep duration is associated with high risk for hypertension. *Sleep* 32(4):491–497.
25. Spiegel K, Tasall E, Penev P and Van Cauter E (2004) Sleep curtailment in healthy young men is associated with decreased leptin levels, elevated ghrelin levels and increased hunger and appetite. *Annals of Internal Medicine* 141(11):846–850.
26. Nguyen N, Varela EJ, Nguyen T *et al.* (2006) Quality of life assessment in the morbidly obese. *Obesity Surgery* 16:531–533.
27. Van Hout GC, Boekestin P, Fortuin FA *et al.* (2006) Psychosocial functioning following bariatric surgery. *Obesity Surgery* 16:787–794.

7. Weight loss surgery: the facts and figures

1. Welbourn R, Fiennes A, Kinsman R and Walton P (2010) *The United Kingdom National Bariatric Surgery Registry. First Registry Report to March 2010*. Henley on Thames: Dentrite Clinical Systems.
2. Buchwald H and Williams SE (2004) Bariatric surgery worldwide 2003. *Obesity Surgery* 14:1157–1164.
3. National Institute for Health and Clinical Excellence (2007) *Bariatric surgical service for the treatment of people with severe obesity. Commissioning guide: implementing NICE guidance*. Available at www.nice.org.uk/media/87F/65/BariatricSurgeryFINALPlusNewToolUpdates
4. Burton PR and Brown WA (2011) The mechanism of weight loss with laparoscopic adjustable gastric banding: induction of satiety not restriction. *International Review of Obesity* 35:S26–S30.
5. Pournaras DJ and le Roux CW (2010) Ghrelin and metabolic surgery. *International Journal of Peptides* doi: 10.1155/2010/217267.
6. Ochner CN, Gibson C, Shanik M *et al.* (2010) Changes in neurohormonal gut peptides following bariatric surgery. *International Journal of Obesity* 1:14.
7. Burton PR, Brown W, Laurie C *et al.* (2011) Outcomes, satiety and adverse upper gastrointestinal symptoms following laparoscopic adjustable gastric band. *Obesity Surgery* 21(5):574–581.
8. Buchwald H, Avidor Y, Braunwald E *et al.* (2004) Bariatric surgery: a systematic review and meta-analysis. *Journal of the American Medical Association* 292:1724–1737.

9. Van Nieuwenhove Y, Ceelen W, Stockman A *et al.* (2010) Long-term results of a prospective study on laparoscopic adjustable gastric banding for morbid obesity. *Obesity Surgery* 21(5):582–587.

10. Sjöström L, Lindroos A-K, Peltonen M *et al.* (2004) Lifestyle, diabetes and cardiovascular risk factors 10 years after bariatric surgery. *New England Journal of Medicine* 351(26):2683–2693.

11. Thomas H and Agrawal S (2011) Systematic review of same-day laparoscopic adjustable gastric band surgery. *Obesity Surgery* 21(6):805–810.

12. Buchwald H, Avidor Y, Braunwald El *et al.* (2004) Bariatric surgery: a systematic review and meta-analysis. *Journal of the American Medical Association* 292(14):1724–37.

13. Dixon JB, O'Brien PE, Playfair J *et al.* (2008) Adjustable gastric banding and conventional therapy for type 2 diabetes: a randomized controlled trial. *Journal of the American Medical Association* 299:316–323.

14. Hutter MH, Schirmer BD, Jones DB *et al.* (2011) First report from The American College of Surgeons Bariatric Surgery Centre Network. Laparoscopic sleeve gastrectomy has morbidity and effectiveness positioned between the band and the bypass. *Annals of Surgery* 254(3):410–420.

15. Cadiere G-B, Himpens J, Bazi M *et al.* (2011) Are laparoscopic gastric bypass after gastroplasty and primary laparoscopic gastric bypass similar in terms of results? *Obesity Surgery* 21(6):692–698.

16. Shi X, Karmali S, Sharma AM *et al.* (2010) A review of laparoscopic sleeve gastrectomy for morbid obesity. *Obesity Surgery* 20:1171–1177.

17. Gill RS, Birch DW, Shi X *et al.* (2010) Sleeve gastrectomy and type 2 diabetes mellitus: a systematic review. *Surgery for Obesity and Related Metabolic Disorders* 6(5):707–713.

18. Bobowicz M, Lehmann A, Orlowski M *et al.* (2011) Preliminary outcomes 1 year after laparoscopic sleeve gastrectomy based on bariatric analysis and reporting outcome system (BAROS). *Obesity Surgery* 21(12):1843–1848.

19. Buchwald H, Estok R, Fahrbach K *et al.* (2009) Weight and type 2 diabetes after bariatric surgery: systematic review and meta-analysis. *American Journal of Medicine* 122(3):248–256.

20. Pournaras DJ, Footitt D, Mahon D and Welbourn R (2011) Reduced phenytoin levels in an epileptic patient following Roux-en-Y gastric bypass for obesity. *Obesity Surgery* 21(5):684–685.

21. Magee CJ, Barry J, Brocklehurst J *et al.* (2011) Outcome of laparoscopic duodenal switch for morbid obesity. *British Journal of Surgery* 98(1):79–84.

22. Scopinaro N, Marinari GM, Camerini GB *et al.* (2005) Specific effects of biliopancreatic diversion on the major components of metabolic syndrome. *Diabetes Care* 28(10):2406–2411.

23. Hedberg J, Hedenström H, Karlsson FA *et al.* (2011) Gastric emptying and postprandial PYY response after biliopancreatic diversion with duodenal switch. *Obesity Surgery* 21(5):609–615.

24. Balsa JA, Botello-Carretero JI, Gomez-Martin JM *et al.* (2011) Copper and zinc serum levels after derivative bariatric surgery: differences between Roux-en-Y gastric bypass and biliopancreatic diversion. *Obesity Surgery* 21(6):744–750.

25. Elliot K (2003) Nutritional considerations after bariatric surgery. *Critical Care Nursing Quarterly* 26(2):133–138.

26. Chelsea & Westminster Hospital NHS Foundation Trust (2009) Bariatric (obesity) surgery: information for patients. Available from www.chelwest. nhs.uk/services/surgery/weightloss

27. Farina MG, Baratta R, Nigro A et al. (2011) Intragastric balloon in association with lifestyle and/or pharmacotherapy in the long-term management of obesity. Obesity Surgery doi: 10.1007/s11695-011-0514-y.

28. Imaz I, Martinez-Cevell C, Garcia-Alvarez EE et al. (2008) Safety and effectiveness of the intragastric balloon for obesity. A meta-analysis. Obesity Surgery 18(7):841–846.

29. Fernandes MAP, Atallah ÁN, Soares B et al. (2007) Intragastric balloon for obesity. Cochrane Database of Systematic Reviews 2007, Issue 1.

30. National Institute for Health and Clinical Excellence (2006) CG43 Obesity: Guidance on the prevention, identification, assessment and management of overweight and obesity in adults and children. Quick reference guide 2 for the NHS. www.nice.org.uk.

8. 'Pressing the re-set button': life after weight loss surgery

1. Bocchieri LE, Meana M and Fisher BL (2002b) Perceived psychosocial outcomes of gastric bypass surgery: a qualitative study. Obesity Surgery 12:781–788.

2. Ogden J, Clementi C, and Aylwin S (2006) The impact of obesity surgery and the paradox of control: a qualitative study. Psychology & Health 21(2):273–293.

3. Odom J, Zalesin KC, Washington TL et al. (2010) Behavioral predictors of weight regain after bariatric surgery. Obesity Surgery 20:349–356.

4. Times Magazine (2011) Suddenly skinny, sexy and confused. 4th March.

5. Ogden J, Avenell S and Ellis G (2011) Negotiating control: patients' experiences of unsuccessful weight-loss surgery. Psychology & Health 26(7): 949–964.

6. Karmali S, Stoklossa CJ, Sharma A et al. (2010) Bariatric surgery: a primer. Canadian Family Physician 56:873–879.

7. Slater GH, Ren CJ, Siegel N et al. (2004) Serum fat-soluble vitamin deficiency and abnormal calcium metabolism after malabsorptive bariatric surgery. Journal of Gastrointestinal Surgery 8:48–55.

8. Tremblay MS, Warburton DER, Janssen I et al. (2011) New Canadian physical activity guidelines. Applied Physiology, Nutrition and Metabolism 36:36–46.

9. Bond DS, Phelan S, Wolfe LG et al. (2008) Becoming physically active after bariatric surgery is associated with improved weight loss and health-related quality of life. Obesity 70:811–814.

10. Livhits M, Mercado C and Yermilov I (2010) Exercise following bariatric surgery: systematic review. Obesity Surgery 20:657–665.

11. Bueter M, Thalheimer A, Lager C et al. (2007) Who benefits from gastric banding? Obesity Surgery 17:1608–1613.

12. Chevallier JM, Paita M, Rodde-Dunet MH et al. (2007) Predictive factors of outcome after gastric banding: a nationwide survey on the role of center activity and patients' behaviour. Annals of Surgery 246:1034–1039.

13. Bond DS, Phelan S, Wolfe LG et al. (2009) Becoming physically active after bariatric surgery is associated with improved weight loss and health-related quality of life. Obesity (Silver Spring) 17:78–83.
14. Rosenberg PH, Henderson KE, White MA et al. (2011) Physical activity in gastric bypass patients: associations with weight loss and psychosocial functioning at 12-month follow up. Obesity Surgery 21(10):1564–1569.
15. Forbush SW, Nof L, Echtermach J and Hill C (2011) Influence of activity on quality of life scores after RYGBP. Obesity Surgery 21(8):1296.
16. Bond DS, Jakicic JM, Unick JL et al. (2010) Pre- to postoperative physical activity changes in bariatric surgery patients: self report vs. objective measures. Obesity 18:2395–2397.
17. Hu FB, Leitzmann MF, Stampfer MJ et al. (2003) Television viewing and other sedentary behaviors in relation to risk of obesity and type 2 diabetes mellitus in women. Journal of the American Medical Association 289:1785–1791.
18. Dunstan DW, Barr ELM, Healy GN et al. (2010) Television viewing time and mortality: the Australian Diabetes, Obesity and Lifestyle Study (AusDiab). Circulation 121:384–391.
19. WeightConcern.org.uk ⏷ www.weightconcern.com/node/119.
20. Ross R, Dagnone D, Jones PJ et al. (2000) Reduction in obesity and related comorbid conditions after diet-induced weight loss in men. A randomized, controlled trial. Annals of Internal Medicine 133:92–103.
21. Cook CM and Edwards C (1999) Success habits of long-term gastric bypass patients. Obesity Surgery 9:80–82.
22. Funnell MM, Anderson RM and Ahroni JH (2005) Empowerment and self-management after weight loss surgery. Obesity Surgery 15:417–422.
23. Elkins G, Whitfield P, Marcus J et al. (2005) Noncompliance with behavioural recommendations following bariatric surgery. Obesity Surgery 15: 546–551.
24. Sjöström L, Lindroos A-K, Peltonen M et al. (2004) Lifestyle, diabetes and cardiovascular risk factors 10 years after bariatric surgery. New England Journal of Medicine 351(26):2683–2693.
25. Wood W and Neal DT (2009) The habitual consumer. Journal of Consumer Psychology 19:579–592.
26. Quinn JM, Pascoe AT, Wood W and Neal DT (2009) Can't control yourself? Monitor those bad habits. Personality and Social Psychology Bulletin 36(4):499–511.
27. Knauper B, McCollam A, Rosen-Brown A et al. (2011) Fruitful plans: adding targeted mental imagery to implementation intentions increases fruit consumption. Psychology and Health http://dx.doi.org.10.1080/08870441003.
28. Webb TL, Sheeran P, Totterdell P et al. (2010) Using implementation intentions to overcome the effect of mood on risky behaviour. The British Journal of Social Psychology http://www.ncbi.nlm.nih.gov/pubmed/21050527.
29. Wansink B and Sobal J (2007) Mindless eating: the 200 daily food decisions we overlook. Environment and Behavior 39(1):106–123.
30. Muraven M and Baumeister RF (2000). Self-regulation and depletion of limited resources: does self-control resemble a muscle? Psychological Bulletin 126:247–259.

31. Orth WS, Madan AK, Taddeucci RJ *et al.* (2008) Support group meeting attendance is associated with better weight loss. *Obesity Surgery* 18(4): 391–394.
32. Livhits M, Mercado LM, Yerilov I *et al.* (2011) Is social support associated with greater weight loss after bariatric surgery? A systematic review. *Obesity Reviews* 12(2):142–148.
33. Sabbioni MEE, Dickson MH, Eychmuller S *et al.* (2002) Immediate results of health related quality of life after vertical banded gastroplasty. *International Journal of Obesity* 26:277–280.
34. Steinberg D and Dryden W (1996) *How to stick to a diet*. London: Sheldon Press.

9. 'It's the best decision I ever made': success stories with weight loss surgery

1. Odom J, Zalesin KC, Washington TL *et al.* (2010) Behavioural predictors of weight regain after bariatric surgery. *Obesity Surgery* 20:349–356.
2. Sjöström L, Lindroos A-K, Peltonen M *et al.* (2004) Lifestyle, diabetes and cardiovascular risk factors 10 years after bariatric surgery. *New England Journal of Medicine* 351(26):2683–2693.
3. Padwal R, Klarenbach S, Wiebe N, *et al.* (2011) Bariatric surgery: a systematic review of the clinical and economic evidence. *Journal of General Internal Medicine* 26(10):1183–1194.
4. Horton ES (2009) Effects of lifestyle changes to reduce risks from diabetes and associated cardiovascular risks: results from large-scale efficacy trials. *Obesity (Silver Spring)* 17(3):S43–48.
5. Welbourn R, Fiennes A, Kinsman R and Walton P (2011) *The United Kingdom National Bariatric Surgery Registry. First Registry Report to March 2010*. Henley on Thames: Dentrite Clinical Systems.
6. Buchwald H, Estok R, Fahrbach K *et al.* (2009) Weight and type 2 diabetes after bariatric surgery: systematic review and meta-analysis. *American Journal of Medicine* 122(3):248–256.
7. Hutter MH, Schirmer BD, Jones DB *et al.* (2011) First report from The American College of Surgeons Bariatric Surgery Centre Network. Laparoscopic sleeve gastrectomy has morbidity and effectiveness positioned between the band and the bypass. *Annals of Surgery* 254(3):410–420.
8. Scopinaro N, Marinari GM, Camerini GB *et al.* (2005) Specific effects of biliopancreatic diversion on the major components of metabolic syndrome. *Diabetes Care* 28(10):2406–2411.
9. Gill RS, Birch DW, Shi X *et al.* (2010) Sleeve gastrectomy and type 2 diabetes mellitus: a systematic review. *Surgery for Obesity and Related Metabolic Disorders* 6(5):707–713.
10. Pournaras DJ, Osborne A, Hawkins SC *et al.* (2010) Remission of type 2 diabetes after gastric bypass and banding. *Annals of Surgery* 252(6):966–971.
11. Deitel M (2011) Update: why diabetes does not resolve in some patients after bariatric surgery. *Obesity Surgery* 21(6):794–796.
12. Peltonen M, Lindroos AK and Torgenseon (2003) Musculoskeletal pain in the obese: a comparison with the general population and long-term changes after conventional and surgical obesity treatment. *Pain* 104:549–557.

13. Suter M, Calmes J-M, Paroc A et al. (2009) Results of Roux-en-Y gastric bypass in morbidly obese vs super-obese patients. *Archives of Surgery* 144(4):312–318

14. Mummadi RR, Kasturi KS, Sood G. (2007) Effect of bariatric surgery on nonalcoholic fatty liver disease (NAFLD): a meta-analysis. *Hepatology* 46(4):294.

15. Smith SC, Edwards CB, Goodman GN et al. (1997) Symptomatic and clinical improvement in morbidly obese patients with gastroesophageal reflux disease following Roux-en-Y gastric bypass. *Obesity Surgery* 7(6):479–484.

16. Pontiroli AE and Morabito A (2011) Long-term prevention of mortality in morbid obesity through bariatric surgery. A systematic review and meta-analysis of trials performed with gastric banding and gastric bypass. *Annals of Surgery* 253 (3):484–487.

17. Adams TD, Gress RE, Smith SC et al. (2007) Long-term mortality after gastric bypass surgery. *New England Journal of Medicine* 357(8): 753–761.

18. Sjöström L, Narbro K, Sjöström CD et al. (2007) Effects of bariatric surgery on mortality in Swedish obese subjects. *New England Journal of Medicine* 357:741–752.

19. Sjöström L, Peltonen M, Jacobson P et al. (2012) Bariatric surgery and long-term cardiovascular events. *Journal of the American Medical Association* 307(1):56–65.

20. Maciejewski ML, Livingston EH, Smith VA et al. (2011) Survival among high-risk patients after bariatric surgery. *Journal of the American Medical Association* 305(23):2419–2426.

21. Maggard MA, Yermilov I, Zhaopiong L et al. (2008) Pregnancy and fertility following bariatric surgery: a systematic review. *Journal of the American Medical Association* 300(19):2286–2296.

22. Dell'Agnolo CM, de Barros Carvalho MD and Pelloso SM (2011) Pregnancy after bariatric surgery: implications for mother and newborn. *Obesity Surgery* 21(6):699–706.

23. De Zwaan M, Lancaster KL, Mitchell JE et al. (2002) Health related quality of life in morbidly obese patients: effect of gastric bypass surgery. *Obesity Surgery* 12:773–780.

24. O'Brien PE, Dixon JB, Laurie C et al. (2006) Treatment of mild to moderate obesity with laparoscopic adjustable gastric banding or an intensive medical program. *Annals of Internal Medicine* 144:625–633.

25. Nguyen NT, Goldman C, Rosenquist J et al. (2001) Laparoscopic versus open gastric bypass: a randomized study of outcomes, quality of life, and costs. *Annals of Surgery* 234:279–289.

26. Nickel MK, Loew TH and Bachler E (2007) Change in mental symptoms in extreme obesity patients after gastric banding part II: six-year follow-up. *International Journal of Psychiatry in Medicine* 37(1):69–79.

27. Ogden J, Clementi C, Aylwin S and Patel A (2005) Exploring the impact of obesity surgery on patient's health status: a quantitative and qualitative study. *Obesity Surgery* 15:266–272.

28. Helmio M, Salminen P, Sintonen H et al. (2011) A 5-year prospective quality of life analysis following laparoscopic adjustable gastric banding for morbid obesity. *Obesity Surgery* 21(10):1585.

29. Canetti L, Berry EM and Elizur Y (2009) Psychosocial predictors of weight loss and psychological adjustment following bariatric surgery and a weight loss programme: the mediating role of emotional eating. *International Journal of Eating Disorders* 42(2):109–117.

30. Ogden J, Clementi C and Aylwin S (2006) The impact of obesity surgery and the paradox of control: a qualitative study. *Psychology and Health* 21(2):273–293.

31. Colles SL, Dixon JB and O'Brien PE (2008) Grazing and loss of control related to eating: two high-risk factors following bariatric surgery. *Obesity* 16(3):615–622.

32. Bocchieri-Ricciardi LE, Chen EY, Munoz D *et al.* (2006) Pre-surgery binge eating status: effect on eating behaviour and weight outcome after gastric bypass. *Obesity Surgery* 16:1198–1204.

33. Schultes B, Ernst B, Wilms B *et al.* (2010) Hedonic hunger is increased in severely obese patents and is reduced after gastric bypass surgery. *American Journal of Clinical Nutrition* 92:277–283.

34. Wadden TA and Sarwer DB (2006) Behavioural assessments of candidates for bariatric surgery: a patient-oriented approach. *Obesity (Silver Spring)* 14(2):S53–62.

35. Vage V, Solhaug JH, Viste A *et al.* (2003) Anxiety, depression and health-related quality of life after jejunoileal bypass: a 25-year follow-up study of 20 female patients. *Obesity Surgery* 13: 706–713.

36. Dixon JB, Dixon ME andO'Brien PE (2003) Depression in association with severe obesity: changes with weight loss. *Archives of Internal Medicine* 163:2058–2065.

37. Herpertz S, Kielmann R, Wolf AM *et al.* (2004) Do psychosocial variables predict weight loss or mental health after obesity surgery? A systematic review. *Obesity Research* 12:1554–1569.

38. Karlsson J, Sjöström L and Sullivan M (1998) Swedish obese subjects (SOS): an intervention study of obesity: two year follow-up of health related quality of life (HRQL) and eating behaviour after gastric surgery for severe obesity. *International Journal of Obesity* 22:113–126.

39. Adami GF, Gandolfo P, Campostano A *et al.* (1998) Body image and body weight in obese patients. *International Journal of Eating Disorders* 24: 299–306.

40. Applegate KL, Friedman KE and Grant JP (2006) Assessments of relationship satisfaction and stability one year after weight loss surgery: a prospective study. Cited in Applegate and Friedman (2008).

41. Sarwer DB, Wadden TA and Fabricatore AN (2005) Psychosocial and behavioural aspects of bariatric surgery. *Obesity Research* 13: 639–648.

42. Goble L, Rand CS and Kuldau JM (1986) Understanding marital relationships following obesity surgery. *Family Therapy* 13:195–202.

43. Woodard GA, Encarnacion B, Pereza *et al.* (2011) Halo effect for bariatric surgery: collateral weight loss in patients' family members. *Archives of Surgery* 146(10):1185–1190.

44. Madan AK, Turham KA and Tichansky DS (2005) Weight changes in spouses of gastric bypass patients. *Obesity Surgery* 15:191–194.

45. Kinzl JF, Traweger C, Trefalt E and Biebl W (2003) Psychosocial consequences of weight loss following gastric banding for morbid obesity. *Obesity Surgery* 13:105–110.

46. Camps M, Zervos E, Goode S and Rosemurgy AS (1996) Impact of bariatric surgery on body image perception and sexuality in morbidly obese patients and their partners. *Obesity Surgery* 6:356–360.

47. Rand CS and MacGregor AM (1991) Successful weight loss following obesity surgery and the perceived liability of morbid obesity. *International Journal of Obesity* 15:577–579.

48. Herpertz S, Kielmann R, Wolf AM *et al.* (2003) Does obesity surgery improve psychosocial functioning? A systematic review. *International Journal of Obesity* 27:1300–1314.

49. Polivy J and Herman CP (2002) If at first you don't succeed: false hopes of self-change. *American Psychologist* 57:677–689. Cited in Wood W and Neal DT (2009) The habitual consumer. *Journal of Consumer Psychology* 19: 579–592.

50. Prochaska JO and DiClemente CC (1992) *Stages of Change in the Modification of Problem Behaviors.* Newbury Park, CA: Sage.

51. Larimer ME, Palmer RS and Marlatt GA (1999) Relapse prevention: an overview of Marlatt's cognitive-behavioral model. *Alcohol Research and Health*. Available at www.thegoalgroup.co.uk/pdf/Relapse%20Prevention.pdf.

52. Bandura A (1977) Self-efficacy: toward a unifying theory of behavioural change. *Psychological Review* 84(2):191–215.

53. Gilbert P (2009) *The Compassionate Mind*. London: Constable & Robinson. A detailed handout outlining the principles of compassionate mind training, *Training our minds in, with and for compassion: an introduction to concepts and compassion-focussed exercises* (Paul Gilbert and colleagues, 2010) can be accessed at www.compassionatemind.co.uk/resources.

54. Steinberg D and Dryden W (1996) *How to Stick to a Diet*. London: Sheldon Press.

10. 'I thought if I was slim the world would be some kind of fairy tale': the risks and challenges of weight loss surgery

1. Cowan GSM (1998) What do patients, families and society expect from the bariatric surgeon? *Obesity Surgery* 8:77–85.

2. Welbourn R, Fiennes A, Kinsman R and Walton P (2010) *The United Kingdom National Bariatric Surgery Registry. First Registry Report to March 2010*. Henley on Thames: Dentrite Clinical Systems.

3. Hutter MH, Schirmer BD, Jones DB *et al.* (2011) First report from The American College of Surgeons Bariatric Surgery Centre Network. Laparoscopic sleeve gastrectomy has morbidity and effectiveness positioned between the band and the bypass. *Annals of Surgery* 254(3): 410–420.

4. The Longitudinal Assessment of Bariatric Surgery (LABS) Consortium (2009) Perioperative safety in the Longitudinal Assessment of Bariatric Surgery. *New England Journal of Medicine* 361(5):445–454.

5. Smith MD, Patterson E, Wahed AS *et al.* (2011) Thirty-day mortality after bariatric surgery: independently adjudicated causes of death in the Longitudinal Assessment of Bariatric Surgery. *Obesity Surgery* 21(11): 1687–1692.

6. Shi X, Karmali S, Sharma AM *et al.* (2010) A review of laparoscopic sleeve gastrectomy for morbid obesity. *Obesity Surgery* 20:1171–1177.

7. Buchwald H, Avidor Y, Braunwald E *et al.* (2004) Bariatric surgery: a systematic review and meta-analysis. *Journal of the American Medical Association* 292:1724–1737.

8. DeMaria EJ, Portenier D and Wolfe L (2007) Obesity surgery mortality risk score: proposal for a clinically useful score to predict mortality risk in patients undergoing gastric bypass. *Surgery for Obesity and Related Diseases* 3(2):134–140.

9. De Maria EJ, Pate V, Warhen M and Winegar DA (2010) Baseline data from the American Society for Metabolic and Bariatric Surgery – designated bariatric surgery centres of excellence using the Bariatric Outcomes Longitudinal Database. *Surgery for Obesity and Related Diseases* 6:347–355.

10. Magee CJ, Barry J, Brocklehurst J *et al.* (2011) Outcome of laparoscopic duodenal switch for morbid obesity. *British Journal of Surgery* 98(1):79–84.

11. Hamdan K, Somers S and Chand M (2011) Management of late postoperative complications of bariatric surgery. *British Journal of Surgery* 98:1345–1355.

12. Sarela AI, Dexter SPL and McMahon MJ (2011) Use of the Obesity Surgery Mortality Risk Score to predict complications of laparoscopic bariatric surgery. *Obesity Surgery* 21(11): 1698–1703.

13. National Institute for Health and Clinical Excellence (2006) *CG43 Obesity: Guidance on the prevention, identification, assessment and management of overweight and obesity in adults and children.* Quick reference guide 2 for the NHS. www.nice.org.uk.

14. Spaw AT and Husted JD (2005) Bleeding after laparoscopic gastric bypass: case report and literature review. *Surgery for Obesity and Related Diseases* 1(2):99–103.

15. Papavramidis ST, Eleftheriadis EE, Papavramidis TS *et al.* (2004) Endoscopic management of gastrocutaneous fistula after bariatric surgery by using a fibrin sealant. *Gastrointestinal Endoscopy* 59(2):296–300.

16. Lewis CE, Jensen C, Tejirian T *et al.* (2009) Early jejunojejunostomy obstruction after laparoscopic gastric bypass: case studies and treatment algorithm. *Surgery for Obesity and Related Diseases* 5(2):203–207.

17. Tarantino I, Warschkow R, Steffen T *et al.* (2011) Is routine cholecystectomy justified in severely obese patients undergoing a laparoscopic Roux-en-Y gastric bypass procedure? A comparative cohort study. *Obesity Surgery* 21(12):1870–1878.

18. Suter M, Calmes JM, Paroz A *et al.* (2006) A 10-year experience with laparoscopic gastric banding for morbid obesity: high long-term complication and failure rates. *Obesity Surgery* 16:829–835.

19. Lancaster RT and Hutter MM (2008) Bands and bypasses: 30-day morbidity and mortality of bariatric surgical procedures as assessed by prospective, multi-center, risk-adjusted ACS-NSQIP data. *Surgical Endoscopy* 22: 2554–2563.

20. Khourseed MA, AlBader IA, Al-Asfar FA *et al.* (2011) Revision of failed bariatric procedures to Roux-en-Y gastric bypass (RYGB). *Obesity Surgery* 21(8):1157.

21. Mitchell JE, Lancaster KL, Burgard MA *et al.* (2001) Long-term follow-up of patients' status after gastric bypass. *Obesity Surgery* 11:464–468.
22. The Hormone Foundation (2010) *The Hormone Foundation's patient guide to endocrine and nutritional management after bariatric surgery.* Available at www.hormone.org/Resources/upload/Post-bariatric-Surgery.
23. Wadden TA, Sarwer DB, Fabricatore AN *et al.* (2007) Psychosocial and behavioural status of patients undergoing bariatric surgery: what to expect before and after surgery. *Medical Clinics of North America* 91:451–469.
24. Chelsea & Westminster Hospital NHS Foundation Trust (2009) *Bariatric (obesity) surgery: information for patients.* Available from www.chelwest. nhs.uk/services/surgery/weightloss.
25. Ogden J, Clementi C, and Aylwin S (2006) The impact of obesity surgery and the paradox of control: a qualitative study. *Psychology & Health* 21(2):273–293.
26. Kushner R, Gleason B and Shanta-Retelny V (2004) Re-emergence of pica following gastric bypass surgery for obesity: a new presentation of an old problem. *Journal of the American Dietetic Association* 104:1393–1397.
27. Brust JCM (2007) Nutrition and alcohol-related neurologic disorders. In L Goldman and D Ausiello (eds) *Cecil medicine* 23rd edn. Philadelphia, PA: Saunders Elsevier.
28. Elliot K (2003) Nutritional considerations after bariatric surgery. *Critical Care Nursing Quarterly* 26(2):133–138.
29. Aasheim ET (2008) Wernicke encephalopathy after bariatric surgery: a systematic review. *Annals of Surgery* 248(5):714–720.
30. *Times Magazine* (2011) *Suddenly skinny, sexy and confused*, 28 January 2011.Accessed at www.streamline-surgical.com/downloads/Saturday-Times-28.01.11.pdf
31. Schrader G, Stefanovic S, Gibbs A *et al.* (1990) Do psychosocial factors predict weight loss following gastric surgery for obesity? *Australian and New Zealand Journal of Psychiatry* 24(4):496–499.
32. Walfish S (2004) Self-assessed emotional factors contributing to increased weight gain in pre-surgical bariatric patients. *Obesity Surgery* 14:1402–1405.
33. Herpertz S, Kielmann R, Wolf AM *et al.* (2004) Do psychosocial variables predict weight loss or mental health after obesity surgery? A systematic review. *Obesity Research* 12:1554–1569.
34. Valley V and Grace DM (1987) Psychosocial risk factors in gastric surgery for obesity: identifying guidelines for screening. *International Journal of Obesity* 11:105–113.
35. Powers PS, Boyd F, Blair CR *et al.* (1992) Psychiatric issues in bariatric surgery. *Obesity Surgery* 2:315–325.
36. Sarwer DB, Wadden TA, Fabricatore AF (2005) Psychosocial and behavioural aspects of bariatric surgery. *Obesity Research* 13:639–648.
37. Adams TD, Gress RE, Smith SC *et a.l* (2007) Long-term mortality after gastric bypass surgery. *New England Journal of Medicine* 357(8) 753–761.
38. Tindle HA, Omalu B, Courcoulas A *et al.* (2010) Risk of suicide after long-term follow-up from bariatric surgery. *American Journal of Medicine* 123(11):1036–1042.

39. Wendling A and Wudyka A (2011) Narcotic addiction following gastric bypass surgery. *Obesity Surgery* 21(5):680–683.

40. Ogden J, Avenell S and Ellis G (2011) Negotiating control: patients' experiences of unsuccessful weight-loss surgery. *Psychology & Health* 26(7):949–964.

41. Applegate KL and Friedman KE (2008) The impact of weight loss surgery on romantic relationships. *Bariatric Nursing and Surgical Patient Care* 3(2):135–141.

42. Sogg S and Gorman MJ (2008) Interpersonal changes and challenges after weight loss surgery. *Primary Psychiatry* 15:61–66.

43. Adams CE, Myers VH, Barbera BL *et al.* (2011) The role of fear of negative evaluation in predicting depression and quality of life four years after bariatric surgery in women. *Psychology* 2(3):150–154.

44. Clark M, Hanna B, Mai J *et al.* (2007) Sexual abuse survivors and psychiatric hospitalization after bariatric surgery. *Obesity Surgery* 17:465–469.

45. Sjöström L, Lindroos AK, Peltonen M *et al.* (2004) Swedish Obese Subjects Study Scientific Group: lifestyle, diabetes and cardiovascular risk factors 10 years after bariatric surgery. *New England Journal of Medicine* 351:2683–2693.

46. Rabner JG and Greenstein RJ (1991) Obesity surgery: expectation and reality. *International Journal of Obesity* 15:841–845.

47. Funnell MM, Anderson RM and Ahroni JH (2005) Empowerment and self-management after weight loss surgery. *Obesity Surgery* 15:417–422.

48. Halverson JD and Koehler RE (1981) Gastric bypass: analysis of weight loss and factors determining success. *Surgery* 90:446–455.

49. Ogden J, Clementi C, Aylwin S and Patel A (2005) Exploring the impact of obesity surgery on patients' health status: a quantitative and qualitative study. *Obesity Surgery* 15:266–272.

50. Colles SL, Dixon JB and O'Brien PE (2008) Grazing and loss of control related to eating: two high-risk factors following bariatric surgery. *Obesity* 16(3):615–622.

51. Karmali S, Stoklossa CJ, Sharma A *et al.* (2010) Bariatric surgery: a primer. *Canadian Family Physician* 56:873–879.

52. Kalarchian MA, Marcus MD, Wilson GT *et al.* (2002) Binge eating among gastric bypass patients at long-term follow-up. *Obesity Surgery* 12: 270–275.

53. Saunders R (2004) 'Grazing': a high risk behaviour. *Obesity Surgery* 14:98–10.

54. Scholtz S, Bidlake L, Morgan J *et al.* (2007) Long-term outcomes following laparoscopic adjustable gastric banding: preoperative psychological sequelae predict outcome at 5-year follow-up. *Obesity Surgery* 17(9): 1220–1225.

55. Canetti L, Berry EM and Elizur Y (2009) Psychosocial predictors of weight loss and psychological adjustment following bariatric surgery and a weight loss programme: the mediating role of emotional eating. *International Journal of Eating Disorders* 42(2):109–117.

56. White MA, Kalarchian MA, Masheb RM *et al.* (2010) Loss of control over eating predicts outcomes in bariatric surgery patients: a prospective, 24-month follow-up study. *Journal of Clinical Psychiatry* 71:175–184.

57. Segal A, Kussunoki DK and Larino MA (2004) Post-surgical refusal to eat: anorexia nervosa, bulimia nervosa or a new eating disorder? A case series. *Obesity Surgery* 14:353–360.
58. Christou NV, Look D and McClean LD (2006) Weight gain after short- and long-limb gastric bypass inpatients followed for longer than 10 years. *Annals of Surgery* 244(5):734–740.
59. Biorserud C, Olbers T and Olsen MF (2011) Patients' experience of surplus skin after laparoscopic gastric bypass. *Obesity Surgery* 21:273–277.
60. Gusenoff JA, Messing S, O'Malley W *et al.* (2008) Temporal and demographic factors influencing the desire for plastic surgery after gastric bypass surgery. *Plastic and Reconstructive Surgery* 121(6):2120–2126.
61. Colwell AS (2010) Current concepts in post-bariatric body contouring. *Obesity Surgery* 20:1178–1182.
62. Nemerofsky RB, Oliak DA and Capella JF (2006) Body lift: an account of 200 consecutive cases in the massive weight loss patient. *Plastic & Reconstructive Surgery* 117(2):414–430.
63. Highton L, Ekwobi C and Rose V (2011) Post-bariatric surgery body contouring in the NHSA – a survey of UK bariatric surgeons. *Journal of Plastic, Reconstructive and Aesthetic Surgery.* http://dx.doi.org/10.1016/j.bjps.2011.09.047
64. Burton PR, Brown W, Laurie C *et al.* (2010) Outcomes, satiety and adverse upper gastrointestinal symptoms following laparoscopic adjustable gastric band. *Obesity Surgery* 21(5):574–581.

11. Taking control: FAQs and resources

1. National Institutes of Health (1998) *Clinical guidelines on the identification, evaluation, and treatment of overweight and obesity in adults: the evidence report.* NIHG Publ. N°. 98-9043. Bethesda, MD: National Institutes of Health.
2. Martins C, Strommen M, Stavne OA *et al.* (2011) Bariatric surgery versus lifestyle interventions for morbid obesity – changes in body weight, risk factors and comorbidities at 1 year. *Obesity Surgery* 21(7):841–849.
3. Avenell A, Broom J, Brown TJ *et al.* (2004) Systematic review of the long-term effects and economic consequences of treatments for obesity and implications for health improvement. *Health Technology Assessment* 8(21).
4. Horton ES (2009) Effects of lifestyle changes to reduce risks from diabetes and associated cardiovascular risks: results from large-scale efficacy trials. *Obesity (Silver Spring)* 17(3):S43–48.
5. Mulrow CD, Chiquette E, Angel L *et al.* (2006) Dieting to reduce body weight for controlling hypertension in adults (Cochrane Review). In *The Cochrane Library*, Issue 4, 2006. London: Wiley.
6. Stenius-Aarniala B, Poussa T, Kvarnstrom J *et al.* (2000) Immediate and long-term effects of weight reduction in obese people with asthma: randomised controlled study. *British Medical Journal* 320(7238):827–832.
7. McTigue KM, Harris R, Hemphill B *et al.* (2003) Screening and interventions for obesity in adults: summary of the evidence for the US Preventive Services Task Force. *Annals of Internal Medicine* 139(11):933–949.

8. Parker ED and Folsom AR (2003) Intentional weight loss and incidence of obesity-related cancers: the Iowa Women's Health Study. *International Journal of Obesity and Related Metabolic Disorders* 27(12):1447–1452.

9. Harvie M, Howell A, Vierkant RA *et al.* (2005) Association of gain and loss of weight before and after menopause with risk of postmenopausal breast cancer in the Iowa Women's Health Study. *Cancer Epidemiology, Biomarkers & Prevention* 14:656–661.

10. Williamson DA, Rejeski J, Lang W *et al.* (2009) Impact of a weight management program on health related quality of life in overweight adults with type 2 diabetes. *Archives of Internal Medicine* 169(2):163–171.

11. Stunkard AJ, Stinnet JL and Smoller JW (1986) Psychological and social aspects of the surgical treatment of obesity. *American Journal of Psychiatry* 143:417–429.

12. Scottish Intercollegiate Guidelines Network (2010) *Management of obesity: a national clinical guideline*. Edinburgh: SIGN. Available at http://www.sign.ac.uk/pdf/sign115.pdf.

13. Loveman E, Frampton GK, Shepherd J *et al.* (2011) The clinical effectiveness and cost effectiveness of long-term weight management schemes for adults: a systematic review. *Health Technology Assessment* 15(2):1–182.

14. Brownell KD and Wadden TA (1992) Etiology and treatment of obesity: understanding a serious, prevalent and refractory disorder. *Journal of Consulting and Clinical Psychology* 60:505–517.

15. Wilson GT (1995) Behavioural treatment of obesity: thirty years and counting. *Advances in Behavioural Research and Therapy* 16:31–75.

16. Ogden J (2003) *The Psychology of Eating: from healthy to disordered behaviour*. Oxford: Blackwell.

17. Bryne S (2002) Psychological aspects of weight maintenance and relapse in obesity. *Journal of Psychosomatic Research* 53:1029–1036.

18. Fobi MAL (1993) Operations that are questionable for control of obesity. *Obesity Surgery* 3:197–200.

19. Hernandez TL, Kittelson JM, Law CK *et al.* (2010) Fat redistribution following suction lipectomy: defense of body fat and patterns of restoration. *Obesity* 19:1388–1395.

Index

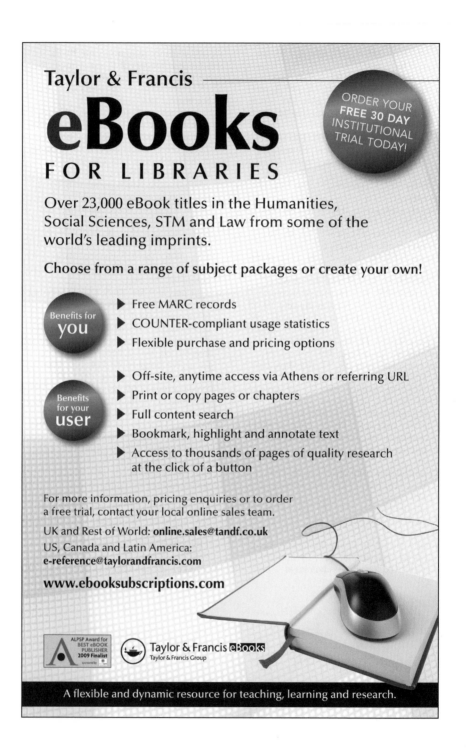